HOW TO SURVIVE MENOPAUSE WITHOUT GOING CRAZY

By Leona Lipari Lee MA, RN

Authors Choice Press
San Jose New York Lincoln Shanghai

How To Survive Menopause Without Going Crazy

All Rights Reserved © 1998, 2001 by Leona Lipari Lee

No part of this book may be reproduced or transmitted in any form or by any means, graphic, electronic, or mechanical, including photocopying, recording, taping, or by any information storage or retrieval system, without the permission in writing from the publisher.

Authors Choice Press
an imprint of iUniverse.com, Inc.

For information address:
iUniverse.com, Inc.
5220 S 16th, Ste. 200
Lincoln, NE 68512
www.iuniverse.com

Originally published by Power Publications

ISBN: 0-595-19241-6

Printed in the United States of America

Dedication:
To all my sisters in menopause especially Liz, Di, Mary, Linda, Barb and Mimi.

—*LLL*

HOW TO SURVIVE MENOPAUSE WITHOUT GOING CRAZY

Table of Contents

1	Introduction	i
1	Mental Health & Menopause: Can Menopause Make You Crazy?	1
2	The Emotional Component of Hot Flashes	11
3	From Mild Anxiety to Full-fledged Panic Attacks	21
4	Depression: Tearfulness, Mood Swings, Just Plain Blahs	29
5	Insomnia & Other Sleep Disturbances	39
6	Impatience: Only One Sign of Irritability	45
7	Forgetfulness	53
8	Fatigue	57
9	Inability to Concentrate	61
10	Creepy-Crawly & Other Weird Happenings	67
11	Fearfulness	75
12	Achieving Good Mental Health During Menopause	83
	References	91

INTRODUCTION

There are moments in our lives when we recognize that we are no longer in control. That somehow we need to find the energy and the courage to do all that is necessary to regain that loss if we are to insure a better quality of life for ourselves. I remember the exact moment this insight hit me. I had been taking hormones for menopausal symptoms for about a year and had received quite a bit of relief from some of the physical problems associated with menopause, particularly menstrual irregularities. However, emotionally I was not myself, and that's putting it mildly. In fact, during the past three or so years prior to my moment of truth, I had changed from a normal, emotionally healthy professional into a tense, tearful, anxiety-ridden wreck of a woman.

On this particular night, when I knew without question that I could no longer go on living the life of an emotional invalid, my husband and I were planning to go out to dinner and a play with friends. I was getting dressed when suddenly I felt as if I was going to die. A "wave" of heat passed through my body. My heart began pounding, I felt weak and disoriented, and believed I was going to pass out at any moment. In the middle of this extremely traumatic emotional experience, the professional side of me thought in amazement, "You're having a panic attack."

I say I was surprised at the realization that I was actually having a panic attack, but I had had a couple of less strong but similar experiences a couple of times in the past, especially in the evenings when we went out. Anxiety was no longer new to me. Not since this whole perplexing thing called menopause began for me.

HOW TO SURVIVE MENOPAUSE
WITHOUT GOING CRAZY

Perimenopause, the two to five years prior to the actual end of a woman's periods, began for me around age 49. And, it started for me the same way it starts for countless other women, with irregular menses. Periods that seemed to never end at times, were either too heavy or nearly nonexistent, that sometimes lasted for three weeks or didn't occur at all for three months. I did what most women do when these changes started happening to me. I saw a doctor. In fact, in the beginning, I ended up seeing three gynecologists, none of whom even mentioned I might be menopausal. When I asked them about the possibility since I had also experienced a couple of barely noticeable hot flashes, two of the three patiently explained to me that the word "menopause" is a Greek derivative and in the literal sense means cessation of menses and because I was still experiencing menes (although very irregular), I was not menopausal. All of these physicians, focusing on one physical symptom, abnormal menstrual periods, rather than a complete physiological and emotional clinical profile, suggested my irregularities might even be due to cancer. One performed an endometrial biopsy, an extremely painful (he said it would be a little uncomfortable) "office D&C" which was negative for cancer cells. But, at a crucial, scary time in my life, three well-intentioned, but not well-informed doctors caused me even greater distress than I was already experiencing.

After about a year of suffering undiagnosed menopausal symptoms, I asked my internist to prescribe a mild antianxiety medication that I had taken in an earlier quest to give up smoking. He gave me the medicine and he also referred me to another gynecologist, who after completing a thorough history and examination, did not hesitate to inform me that I was in the perimenopause stage of life and that I definitely needed to be on hormones. I did not even know that there was a perimenopausal stage that can begin as early as 10 years before actual menopause and that the frightening things that were happening to me are fairly common during this period.

I'd like to be able to say that I started taking estrogen or HRT, hormone replacement therapy, as it is commonly called and I was miraculously cured of all my menopausal woes. That did not happen. According to some experts, hormones can cause a heightened feeling of well-being. Emotionally, I felt a little better, but only a little. At first, the Premarin pills that I took certainly reduced the number and intensity of the hot flashes that were now full-blown after a wasted year of trying to discover what was wrong with me. HRT also helped to alleviate some of the other physical symptoms, vaginal tightness and dryness, frequent urination, and especially the irregular periods that had been occurring for a couple of years.

But, I continued to experience a variety of psychological symptoms that I was not even sure were associated to perimenopause. I was very moody. I had seldom cried before I entered the so-called "Change of Life." Now, I was constantly wiping away tears. I remember in one 24-hour period in particular, I cried because my son was thinking about getting engaged, because I watched "Field of Dreams" for the 20th time, because my favorite football team, the Saints, lost, and because my favorite basketball team, the Spurs, won. Anything could set me off. It didn't matter if it was good or bad news. The tears just kept right on flowing.

Although there were many unusual symptoms that made me wonder if I were indeed going crazy, perhaps the one that was most devastating to me had to do with the extreme feelings of anxiety that became more frequent as time passed. Things got so bad I began keeping a journal. I recorded every episode of anxiety, listed the foods I had eaten, the stresses I was under, what I was doing when they occurred, and what measures I took to get through each one. I kept a journal for many months and discovered that certain foods, some strong smells and loud noises, excitement, and stress were almost always associated with these anxiety attacks. I also discovered that high levels of anxiety was always connected to hot flashes in some way.

I knew that anxiety attacks could lead to phobias and I worried that I might be developing anticipatory anxiety about something as mundane as going out to eat, one of my favorite forms of entertainment. I could sometimes take one of my little anti-anxiety pills, but they often did not work

HOW TO SURVIVE MENOPAUSE
WITHOUT GOING CRAZY

at all. So, these bouts of anxiety became increasingly worrisome to me until that fateful night when I experienced the major panic attack and decided I had a severe, potentially incapacitating problem that I needed to do something about.

That night I did something I had never done before and vowed I would never do again. I made my excuses and canceled my plans for the evening. I felt very embarrassed and frightened by the fact that I could no longer control what was happening to me. This whole affair made me extremely depressed and I promised my husband that I was going to get some help as soon as possible.

I am a registered nurse and have worked in the mental health field for over 20 years and not once in that time have I ever seen a psychiatrist except on a social basis. On the Monday following my "crisis," I called one and made an appointment for the following week. I had never been on the other side of the desk and was extremely uncomfortable. But, I had chosen a woman because I believed she would be more informed in the area of menopause. Was I wrong!

Several of the authorities on menopause believe that how one manages this stage in life is determined by cultural and social factors. They downplay the role of hormone deficiency on severity of symptoms. This psychiatrist was no different. She talked a great deal about the changes in my life. The fact that my children were grown and gone and that we had moved to a different city when my husband was promoted and I was no longer working full time and so on. I tried to help her understand that although these changes had occurred, they had happened years ago and I was extremely happy with my life, with my marriage, with my semi-retirement. We did agree that on the night in question and perhaps a few times before, I had experienced panic attacks and she prescribed the drug of choice for this condition, Xanax. She told me there were little or no side effects except addiction. That was all! I left her office with a prescription for a drug I would never take (the PDR showed three pages of side effects) and another appointment I knew I would not keep, thinking, "Just one more doctor who doesn't know a darn thing about menopause."

Shortly after my disastrous visit to the psychiatrist, my gynecologist called to tell me that despite taking HRT for about a year, my estrogen level was extremely low. He recommended increasing the dosage, but I was hesitatant about taking too much of a drug about which we still know so little. We agreed that I might get better absorption using the patch, so we decided to try that for a while. I say "we" because this physician and I are partners in the treatment of my menopausal symptoms and that's the way it should be for any doctor-patient relationship. Anyway, I continued to have hot flashes with one patch, so we tried two with much better results.

I thought I was going to breeze through menopause like I did through every other stage of my life. I was too busy living to really think about it much at all. That's why I had so much trouble dealing with the changes. I simply did not associate all of the miserable symptoms I was having to what most of the so-called experts led me to believe would be a natural and uneventful change of life that was going to leave me "full of zest."

I began asking questions early on only to learn that there were too few answers on the subject of menopause and practically none on the emotional component of this stage of life. And, when I couldn't get all the answers I needed from the medical profession or from the many books I read as I researched the matter, I began to question my family, friends, neighbors, co-workers, sometimes even perfect strangers about their own menopausal experiences. Many had had hysterectomies in their 30's and 40's, but we soon discovered that although the cause of menopause may be different, the symptoms were the same. A few of my menopausal friends became a much needed support group for me during this period of emotional upheaval. So many of these women whom I questioned early on and those I questioned in a survey for this book experienced many emotional problems during menopause that like myself, they simply were not aware were part of the syndrome and had not the slightest idea how to cope with them.

I decided to write this book for them and for others who must somehow

HOW TO SURVIVE MENOPAUSE
WITHOUT GOING CRAZY

with very little help, learn to cope with what I have come to think of as the "nesses" of menopause: sadness, nervousness, weariness, tearfulness, breathlessness, sleeplessness, weakness, dizziness, numbness, forgetfulness, tenseness, and perhaps the one that becomes the most incapacitating of all in terms of disrupting one's sense of well-being, fearfulness.

MENTAL HEALTH & MENOPAUSE: CAN MENOPAUSE MAKE YOU CRAZY?

CHAPTER 1

MENTAL HEALTH & MENOPAUSE: CAN MENOPAUSE MAKE YOU CRAZY?

Lyn is an attractive 44-year-old writer who had a hysterectomy at age 35 and who has been taking estrogen ever since. "Once at a party," she writes, "we were doing alliterative farewells. Mine had something about 'many magnificent menopausal maniacs' referring to ourselves. We all laughed deep down - because all of us women knew what it felt like to be maniacal."

Lyn and her friends were joking as women have been doing for ages about the legendary and often frightening connection between menopause and mental health. We love to tell each other stories about someone we knew or heard of who went a little nuts during "The Change" -- like my distant cousin, Emelda, who wore a bright red kerchief on her head and men's socks on her hands and up her arms. When we were kids, my sisters and I spent a lot of time running from Emelda who on her bad days wasn't hesitant to come after us with a beat-up old broom. I remember my mom shaking her head and whispering something about the "change," and telling us she was harmless, but to stay away from her just in case. I don't know if poor Emelda was really going through menopause, but this vivid childhood memory has stayed with me all these years.

Many of the so-called modern day experts are fond of telling us that menopause is a natural stage of life and even the National Institute on Aging

HOW TO SURVIVE MENOPAUSE
WITHOUT GOING CRAZY

in an outdated 1986 pamphlet still available to the public as of this writing, entitled "The Menopause Time of Life" is quick to point out that there are "no specific mental disorders associated with menopause, and research shows that women experience no more depression during these years than at other times during life." Then why, we ask, do so many of us feel depressed? Why are we anxious, irritable, angry, weak?

In a hilarious January, 93 episode of the then popular TV series, Picket Fences, a menopausal woman runs over her husband with a steam roller, killing him. She pleads not guilty by reason of insanity brought on by menopause. In this fictional account, the age-old argument about whether or not menopause can make you crazy was decided legally. The show's heroine was freed after the court decided that she had indeed acted irrationally because she was menopausal. But, this is only fiction, we think as we breathe a sigh of relief and laugh at the absurdity of it all.

In the past, the idea of insanity and menopause was not nearly as far-fetched as it is today. A couple of years ago, a friend of mine was working in a psychiatric hospital that was founded in the early 1830's. The hospital was being renovated at the time, and he told me about an old journal that was found in the midst of the chaos. The discovery was actually a record of admissions to the hospital for the year 1894. It contained the names, ages, reasons for the admissions and the final dispositions for all of the patients. Some of the admit diagnoses such as melancholia, dementia, and mania were not unusual for the times. However, two of the admit diagnoses, "broken heart" and "unrequited love" were surprising and touching and one diagnosis listed for several of the female patients that was especially surprising and of immense interest to me since I was at the height of my own menopausal *crazies* at the time, was "change of life."

When I told another friend about this interesting discovery, she said, "How sad!" Her simple response summed up my own feelings and probably those of all menopausal women who can relate to those poor women. Although the journal did not go into the symptoms these women were experiencing that warranted such drastic action as hospitalization in

MENTAL HEALTH & MENOPAUSE: CAN MENOPAUSE MAKE YOU CRAZY?

an insane asylum, a review of the literature gives us a fairly clear idea of what they were probably going through.

In her well-research book, *The Change: Woman, Aging and the Menopause,* Germaine Greer offers a full account of the early link between menopause and psychiatry. Despite the seriousness of the subject, I was actually amused by one anonymous contributor to an 1851 edition of the *Journal of Psychological Medicine and Mental Pathology* cited by Greer. He describes the cessation of ovarian function as an "unwomanly condition (that) doubtless renders her repulsive to man, while her envious, overbearing temper, renders her offensive to her own sex." Scary, huh?

However, Ms. Greer's overall descriptions of this era and of the humiliations women endured during the frightening period of "climacteric insanity" as one early psychiatrist unfortunately dubbed it, were far from a laughing matter. In 1896, one well-known fore-father of psychiatry, Emil Kraeplin, describes a 54-year-old woman who "complained of heat in her head and uneasiness at her heart, felt weak and excited and was tired of life, especially in the morning." Kraeplin called her condition involutional melancholia. This woman, as Ms. Greer so astutely points out, was probably experiencing an "uncomfortable menopause" which along with other factors "placed her in a madhouse." As my empathetic friend said, "How sad!" How sad indeed! No wonder women dreaded menopause in those days, and no wonder some of that fear remains to this day.

I began my own career as a psychiatric nurse in the mid-sixties and although I do not recall menopausal-related admissions to the psychiatric hospital where I worked, I believe some of the women treated for depression and anxiety may have, in fact, been going through menopause. According to a 1963 revised edition of the 1945 medical book, *Emotional Problems of Living,* O. Spurgeon English, M.D., and Gerald H.J. Pearson, M.D., discuss symptoms of menopause that might "necessitate going to a mental hospital." The authors list mood disturbances such as irritability, depression, remorsefulness, bitterness and pessimism, as well as some physiological symptoms such as "hot flushes, cold shivers, sensations

HOW TO SURVIVE MENOPAUSE
WITHOUT GOING CRAZY

of alternating heat and cold accompanied by perspiration."

It is interesting to note that English and Pearson attribute the mood disturbances to women who have lived "unwisely between the ages of twelve and forty-two and can build up a great many regrets over which to be irritable, depressed, etc." Whatever this means! What is important here is the fact the emotional problems that menopausal women experienced in the 1800's and throughout history that prompted hospitalization still plague us to this day. Yet, the average woman is as ill-informed about and as poorly prepared for this stage of her life as was her counterpart in the early 19th century. We are still baffled by what happens to us emotionally during menopause. We still feel like a Kraeplin case study.

Somewhere along the way, psychiatry seems to have lost interest in the relationship between menopause and mental health. Involutional melancholia was removed from psychiatric diagnostic criteria sometime in the late 70's and depression, at least, was disassociated from its earlier link to menopause. In a 1989 paper, "Psychiatric Syndromes Linked to Reproductive Function in Women: A Review of Current Knowledge", contributed to the *American Journal of Psychiatry*, Michael J. Gitlin, M.D. and Robert O. Pasnau, M.D., discuss the fact that there is little evidence to support depression, at least, as a menopausal "entity." They say "more recent research has seemingly put to rest the time-honored concept of involutional melancholia first delineated by Kraeplin."

It is amazing that over 100 years have gone by since menopause was first discussed in terms of its psychiatric connection, and we are still unclear about that relationship.

According to a 1992 government sponsored background paper, *The Menopause, Hormone Therapy, and Women's Health*, "understanding of the relationships among aging, the menopause, and behavioral change is incomplete... the actual prevalence of minor psychological and somatic symptoms directly related to lowered levels of ovarian estrogen remains speculative at best." The authors of this publication go on to explain that the reason we know so little about these relationships is because many of

MENTAL HEALTH & MENOPAUSE: CAN MENOPAUSE MAKE YOU CRAZY?

the studies have "relied on small samples of self-selected women seeking treatment for symptoms." It's no secret that research on women's issues has been almost non-existent until very recently.

So, in the light of so few scientific women's studies on menopause, and until the results of current studies are made available, who better to go to for our answers about this crucial phase of our lives than the women who have experienced and who are currently experiencing the emotional impact of menopause. We, in essence, are the experts. In the end, it doesn't really matter if there is a scientific name for what we are feeling, although validation of our experiences by medical authority would certainly be welcome. But, by sharing our experiences with each other, we validate for ourselves that what we are experiencing is real, that it is not all in our heads as we are so frequently told, and that although some of our symptoms may differ, there are several that many of us will share in common.

* * * *

Marcie was only 42 years old when she began experiencing symptoms of menopause brought on prematurely by chemotherapy received for breast cancer. Because of the cancer that resulted in a mastectomy, she was unable to take estrogen supplements. As a result, Marcie had suffered years of sometimes "debilitating" problems prior to actual menopause, including depression and anxiety attacks. She believes her emotional state was directly related to some of the life-altering physical symptoms that were occurring. She found relief only after menopause when she no longer suffered "hormonal imbalances". Marcie speaks candidly of this stressful period of her life: "I can bear witness to the fact that these symptoms greatly diminish the quality of life for the individual experiencing them and the people in the life of the person." Marcie's gynecologist knew very little about menopause at the time and was very typical in his inability to provide much help. He has just recently informed her, however, that he has gone back to school, so to speak, attending workshops and seminars about menopause since so many of his patients are now complaining of

HOW TO SURVIVE MENOPAUSE
WITHOUT GOING CRAZY

problems associated with this phase of life. This awareness on her gynecologist's part is encouraging to Marcie, but last month when she received a brochure from her local hospital with the "news" that depression is not related to menopause, she became really angry. So much for Marcie's hoped-for enlightenment of the medical establishment in the 90's.

Marcie and other intelligent, well-informed women like her should be encouraged by a few of the more recently published authorities on menopause. Some are starting to acknowledge an emotional component to the change and once again are *beginning* to discuss, at least, the role of depression and anxiety during this phase of hormonal change. Some of these authors are dedicating whole chapters rather than paragraphs to the issue of mental health and menopause.

Raymond G. Burnett, M.D., in his revised 1987 guide, *Menopause: All Your Questions Answered*, lists the following signs of menopause and the frequency of occurrence:

Irritability	92%
Lethargy/Fatigue	88%
Depression	78%
Headaches	71%
Hot Flashes	68%
Forgetfulness	64%
Weight Gain	61%
Insomnia	51%
Joint Pain/Backache	48%
Palpitations	44%
Crying Spells	42%
Constipation	37%
Burning Upon Urination	20%
Decreased Sexual Drive	20%

Over half of these complaints are directly related and several more are

MENTAL HEALTH & MENOPAUSE: CAN MENOPAUSE MAKE YOU CRAZY?

indirectly related to an emotional component of menopause. Burnett agrees with several of the latest authorites that "low levels of estrogen occurring in the perimenopause years do have a psychological effect on important centers in the brain." He goes on to list depression, irritability, forgetfulness, insomnia, crying spells, lethargy and fatigue as some of the changes we might experience during perimenopause.

In *Managing Your Menopause*, another authority on the subject, Wulf Utian, M.D., Ph.D., also discusses emotional problems associated with menopause. He lists tiredness, sadness, confusion, pessimism, tenseness, headaches, irritability, and slow performance and offers a complete treatment regime as part of his overall Utian Menopause Management Program.

And, in her beautifully written, *The Silent Passage*, Gail Sheehy offers a fairly comprehensive account of depression and its relationship to menopause. She also deals with other emotional facets of menopause such as anxiety, memory loss, nervousness and irritability. Sheehy, like Burnett and Utian, seems to understand the fact that any useful discussion of menopause is not complete unless the undeniably significant emotional component of this life stage is presented.

Finally, in my search for answers to the emotional upheaval of menopause, I came across a comprehensive and timely scientific paper in the Nurses Association of the American College of Obstetricians and Gynecologists (NAACOG) 1991 issue of *Clinical Issues*. This article, "New Perspectives on the Relationship of Hormone Changes to Affective Disorders in the Perimenopause" by Elizabeth Lee Vliet, M.D. and Virginia Lee Hutcheson Davis, M.S., regretfully not readily available to the lay person, gives an excellent account of how the "fluctuations and declines in hormone levels are physiologic changes that may have a significant impact on perimenopausal mood changes."

Can menopause make you crazy? Every bit of evidence available to us today leads us to the conclusion that we will not become psychotic, extremely depressed and/or suicidal, or permanently, severely emotionally

HOW TO SURVIVE MENOPAUSE
WITHOUT GOING CRAZY

or behaviorally handicapped at least to the degree that we'll need to be "put away."

Having shared that encouraging little piece of information on the severity of emotional symptoms during menopause to put your mind at ease, I need to also make you aware of the very real possibility that you will probably experience one or more of the physical, emotional and behavioral symptoms that will at times make you feel as if you are indeed going nuts. In the following chapters, we will concentrate on some of the psychological signs of menopause that the above-mentioned authors have listed as well as some of the lesser known symptoms that other experts have discussed. We will focus on those symptoms that the menopausal women I know and others I have contacted by self-report survey during the writing of this book have indicated as giving them the most trouble.

We will look at hot flashes and the emotional problems associated with them. We will discuss the known causes of anxiety and panic attacks. We will provide a somewhat historical perspective on depression and menopause. Insomnia, and irritability, as well as forgetfulness and fatigue will all be discussed. Some of the lesser acknowledged and understood signs such as difficulty concentrating and the "creepy" skin feeling that many women experience but do not associate with menopause will be explored. And, perhaps the most significant sign of all, fearfulness, will be discussed in terms of how preparation for the emotional and physical changes that may occur can help alleviate the fear associated with menopause in general and what's happening to us specifically.

The most frequently asked question by menopausal women today is "When will it be over?" Most of the emotional symptoms experienced during menopause occur during perimenopause, the 2-5 years prior to the cessation of periods. But, encouragingly, there does exist what I like to call "The other side of menopause." Many women find their symptoms disappear or are greatly diminished by the time they are post menopausal.

Meanwhile, we must get through the traumatic, upheaval of perimenopause as best we can. In the following chapters we will discuss

MENTAL HEALTH & MENOPAUSE: CAN MENOPAUSE MAKE YOU CRAZY?

specific ways to deal with each of the emotional problems listed above. We will also provide a review of past and current treatments and/or solutions to the problems from a holistic approach from hormone replacement to relaxation and imaging techniques to vitamins and exercise. Hopefully, you will learn, as I have, how to conquer your fears and survive menopause without going crazy.

HOW TO SURVIVE MENOPAUSE WITHOUT GOING CRAZY

THE EMOTIONAL COMPONENT OF HOT FLASHES

CHAPTER 2

THE EMOTIONAL COMPONENT OF HOT FLASHES

I remember the first time I had a hot flash in public. I had been working in a pain management clinic for less than a month when I was required to present a case to the treatment team. Since it was the first time I was presenting to this particular team, a group of physicians, psychologists, physical and occupational therapists and social workers, most of whom I had not yet met, I was a little tense to begin with. However, I was well prepared and very familiar with the team setting. I started the presentation as I had done many times before in similar situations with a lot of confidence.

I was not quite halfway through my presentation with about forty eyes focused on my face when I felt a little flutter in my stomach. Delayed nervous reaction, I thought. Then I felt the heat creeping up from my neck to my face. I could only imagine what those twenty or so professionals were seeing . . . a very, very red-faced nurse. The more I imagined what my co-workers were seeing, the more embarrassed I felt, and the more embarrassed I felt, the redder I became. At least, that's what I envisioned.

But what could I do? I certainly couldn't do what my body was telling to do. Strip! The thought kept flashing through my mind. Strip! I could have settled by subtly attempting to fan myself, but that would have only confirmed for my audience that I was indeed in the middle of a menopausal hot flash. So I did the only thing I could do under the

HOW TO SURVIVE MENOPAUSE
WITHOUT GOING CRAZY

circumstances. I did nothing. I simply pretended it wasn't happening. I continued with my presentation as best I could, thinking, "What a nightmare." But, it wasn't a bad dream. It really happened and now they <u>knew</u>. So much for impressing my new co-workers with my professional expertise. In my opinion, I had been reduced to a middle-aged woman at the mercy of my hormones or rather my lack of them. Of course, I never really knew what my co-workers saw that day. No one ever mentioned the incident and I certainly never brought it up. I just know how I perceived what happened and that's what really matters in the case of experiencing hot flashes at inopportune times.

Most women experience hot flashes in the perimenopause phase of life. No one knows the exact number of women who suffer the often embarrassing, nearly always uncomfortable symptom, but latest estimates are that anywhere from 70% to 85% have hot flashes sometime during menopause.

Not only are we still in the dark about how many women actually experience hot flashes, but incredibly we still do not know exactly what causes them. There are three popular theories about why hot flashes occur during menopause: 1. The drop in the estrogen level. 2. Changes in the brain. 3. Dilation of blood vessels. Some scientists believe that these three probable causes of hot flashes are related. That the drop in estrogen levels during menopause triggers the brain's hypothalamus which regulates body temperature to, in turn, trigger the dilation of the blood vessels in the skin.

Also, some authorities like to try to distinguish between the hot flush and the hot flash. And while it's true that first you flash and then you flush, I use the term, hot flash, exclusively when describing this unpleasant menopausal phenomenon. I believe some women experience a flash or warning without becoming red or flushed. And, some women actually experience the flush or reddening of the face and neck without the flash or aura that serves to alert us to prepare for the eminent flush. In order to understand the difference, you need to be aware of what's happening to your body during the hot flash.

THE EMOTIONAL COMPONENT OF HOT FLASHES

Most women will experience a little warning before the actual hot flash. This "aura" or feeling that a hot flash is about to occur may take the form of a small flutter in the pit of your stomach accompanied by feeling slightly anxious or nervous for no apparent reason. Within a couple of minutes, you will begin to feel the rise in your skin temperature. You actually feel the heat rise from your chest to your face and if you look into a mirror during the flash, your face and neck will appear red. Probably not as red as you imagine, but red never-the-less. Next, you may begin to perspire, sometimes slightly, but often profusely. When this happens in the middle of the night, you may even have to change your nightclothes, because the hot flash is more often than not followed by chills as your body fights to right itself. Then you can actually find yourself feeling very cold and clammy. The hot flash may last only a minute or so, the average length of one is about 3 minutes. But some unlucky women may experience them for as long as 30 minutes and even an hour at a time. Some women experience one after another on a daily basis. Some may have them once or twice a week. Others, only once a month. Probably less than 25% never experience hot flashes at all. Not one woman I talked with or surveyed belonged to this elite group of very lucky women.

Menopausal women have been studied while actually experiencing hot flashes so we know certain physiological changes are taking place. For example, although skin temperature actually increases 7 or 8°, body temperature does not rise at all. In fact, after the flash, body temperature actually drops. The heart rate is increased and the finger blood flow is also increased. Blood pressure is also increased. During a hot flash, the hormone epinephrine is increased and the hormone norepinephrine is decreased and this probably accounts for the increased heart rate, blood pressure, and cardiac output. The same "fight or flight" reaction we have in situations of extreme stress or anxiety. Blood levels show other hormones are also increased during and after the hot flash, (luteinizing and adrenal in particular), but no one entirely understands the relationship between these hormones and the hot flash.

HOW TO SURVIVE MENOPAUSE
WITHOUT GOING CRAZY

Is there anything you can do to prevent hot flashes? We do know that certain things may precipitate a flash, so although you may not be able to entirely stave off a flash knowing what can set one off should be helpful. Anything that makes you feel hot is a likely culprit:

1. Hot and spicy or very large meals as well as hot liquids.
2. Very hot baths.
3. Hot weather.
4. Hot room.
5. Warm bed.
6. Too much clothing and/or clothes made from synthetic fibers.
7. Over-exercising or getting over-heated.
8. Alcohol.
9. Stress and/or emotional upsets.

Avoiding the above listed precipitators of hot flashes will help lessen the frequency and severity of them. So you must stay away from the Tabasco, keep the air conditioning and fans humming in the summer and don't overheat your home in the winter. Wear cool cottons and silks and dress in layers so if you do feel the need to strip, you can do so without attracting too much attention. Carry a fan. Sip cool drinks. Throw cold water on your face if you're in a situation where this is feasible. Of course, this could cause havoc with your makeup and could evoke more stares than the hot flash itself. And, more important than anything else, try to avoid stress. Although you can have a hot flash while just sitting quietly, a stressful lifestyle can certainly cause an increase in both the number and severity of hot flashes. Don't feel obligated to engage in stressful activities. Take care of yourself first. I'll discuss the effects of stress on menopause in more detail later, but for now remember that stress is one of the main activators of the dreaded hot flash and cannot be ignored.

* * * *

THE EMOTIONAL COMPONENT OF HOT FLASHES

Joan is a 54-year-old mother of six who began having menopausal symptoms at age 50. She had daily hot flashes sometimes "every few minutes" and became anxious when the flashes began. She experienced night sweats that resulted in insomnia and awakening early on an almost nightly basis. She also started having migraine headaches along with the hot flashes. She was taking hormones at the time, but her overall health began deteriorating and at one point she says she would actually "go into spells" and "did not know people around me." Joan saw a specialist and was taken off the hormones and says both the headaches and the hot flashes disappeared at first, but returned a few months later.

Joan suffered through several years of hot flashes that resulted in the usual accompanying emotional problems such as anxiety and irritability. Whether or not the "spells" she experienced were related to hot flashes is questionable especially since her physician believed they were related to the hormones and because they disappeared once she was taken off them. Other women have complained of rather unusual reactions to hormone replacement and I'll discuss this further later on.

But, what then is the emotional component of hot flashes and is there really one at all? According to the authors of <u>Menopause: A Guide For Women And The Men Who Love Them,</u> "Hot flashes and some degree of emotional distress are common." I have listed those emotional problems usually experienced because of hot flashes. Some are apparent while others are a little more less so:

    1. Embarrassment. You blush. You actually turn red. You may have been able to pass for 10 years younger than your actual age before now. But when other women see those rosy cheeks, the gig is up. You think everyone knows you're menopausal and this belief, although far-fetched, is distressful for most of us.

    2. Fear. Your heart is racing. You can actually hear it beating. You think others can hear it as well. The adrenaline has been released and it's preparing you for a fight ahead, except there is no fight. If you've ever had

HOW TO SURVIVE MENOPAUSE
WITHOUT GOING CRAZY

heart palpitations, you know what it's like. It's scary. You may not associate this experience with your hot flashes and that increases your fear.

3. Insomnia. You lose sleep. Lots of it. You can't get to sleep because you're too hot. Or you wake up at 3a.m. to change your bedclothes and linens because you are drenched with sweat. You are tired the next day and irritable. Very irritable. You can't seem to concentrate. You feel physically and emotionally lousy.

4. Your love life is going down the drain. You adore your spouse or significant other, but the last thing you want when you're in the middle of a hot flash is to be touched by another hot body. Especially if that hot body is wearing wool pajamas, thermal underwear, and a ski cap in order to deal with the fact that it's 36° outside and you still insist on sleeping with the air-conditioning and the ceiling fan on. At a time in your life when you most need cuddling, you simply will opt for feeling cool instead. "I love you", you say, "but, I'll kill you if you touch me." Definitely not the best way to keep the passion in your relationship.

5. You feel anxious just before the flash. This happens so often that you find it affects your self-assurance. Suppose you get so nervous, you pass out. Will this happen during social events you wonder? Like right in the middle of your daughter's wedding? Will I be able to function feeling so anxious? Will I embarrass my family? My friends? The more you worry about being anxious, the more anxious you become. Then you begin to feel depressed about not being able to function as you used to. Thus, an unfortunate cycle may develop that is not at all conducive to good mental health.

* * * *

Roberta is a 62-year-old African-American who looks much older than her stated age. She began having hot flashes when she turned 50 years old. She still has them periodically over 10 years later. When asked if she ever tried hormones, she becomes indignant, as if taking hormones would show weakness on her part. The women in her family do use "herbs" when the flashes get real bad, but mostly they just

THE EMOTIONAL COMPONENT OF HOT FLASHES

tolerate them.

Roberta has chosen not to avail herself of the most effective remedy for hot flashes available today, estrogen. It makes sense to assume that if hot flashes are indeed caused by a lack or decreasing amount of estrogen, then using estrogen replacement therapy (ERT) will indeed get rid of the flashes. I know of not one woman who has taken estrogen for hot flashes who hasn't received some relief from the problem. And, quickly, too. Usually, after only a couple of weeks at the most, no more hot flashes, and even more remarkable, no more night sweats.

So, why do some women choose to suffer this miserable symptom of menopause with estrogen so available? A lot of women, like Roberta, are simply afraid to put a foreign substance into their bodies. Some have heard that estrogen causes breast cancer and, of course, some women like Marcie who have actually had breast cancer, cannot use ERT. Many women have been told that ERT can cause hypertension and won't risk aggravating or developing this condition. Others think estrogen will cause weight gain, a fate most of us are already battling as we age. Some women report side effects from ERT, especially if they're taking progestin along with the estrogen (HRT or hormone replacement therapy). Like Joan, who experienced "spells" during which she didn't recognize loved ones until she was taken off hormones, others have reported what they perceive to be strange side effects. Billie, my golf partner, told me her whole right side was temporarily paralyzed until she was taken off hormones. Many women report increased depression and other PMS type symptoms while on HRT.

The pros and cons of ERT and HRT will be discussed more thoroughly in Chapter 12. There are, however, other methods available to us for the relief of hot flashes. Catapres, a drug sometimes taken to lower blood pressure is sometimes prescribed by physicians. It is said to be only about 40% effective, however. Another antihypertensive drug, Inderal, has also been prescribed to relieve hot flashes. Several other non-hormonal drugs have been used to alleviate hot flashes with varying degrees of success, but none are as effective as estrogen. Among these are Bellergal, which may

HOW TO SURVIVE MENOPAUSE
WITHOUT GOING CRAZY

be habit forming and various tranquilizers to reduce the anxiety associated with the flashes.

Like Roberta, many women choose not to use drugs at all to counteract the discomfort and distress of hot flashes and opt for alternative therapies such as vitamins, especially vitamin E. Most physicians are not yet willing to encourage the use of vitamin E since there is no scientific data to validate its effectiveness. On the other hand, many physicians will tell women to take it if they feel it helps. It's not going to hurt.

Ginseng, an herb, is a natural form of estrogen and is often taken in tea form. However, most professionals caution against the use of ginseng because it is a drug. You never know how much you need and are taking and it has been known to cause high blood pressure.

Exercise and proper diet, sometimes referred to as alternative therapies for hot flashes will be discussed in Chapter 12 in terms of overall effectiveness for menopausal symptoms in general.

As I slowly began my journey to the other side of menopause, I attended my son's wedding in New York City. Even if it had not been held in the middle of July, on the hottest Saturday during the death-threatening heat wave of '93, I would have still suffered. Young adults should marry either before or after their mothers' menopauses, never during. Try to convince your daughters that being a June bride is really not so special. Be sure to keep a straight face when you tell them that winter weddings held outdoors in sub-freezing temperatures can be lovely. You don't need to add how much more accommodating for menopausal moms they also can be.

Needless to say, I could not control the weather during the week I was in the Northeast for the wedding. But, I could control the hot flashes to a certain degree, by monitoring what I wore, what I ate and drank, and by taking several other measures discussed in this chapter. Wearing two estrogen patches (on my doctor's advise) didn't hurt either. I experienced only one of the major hot flashes during this wonderful, but highly stressful and extremely emotional event. And that was after enduring several hours

THE EMOTIONAL COMPONENT OF HOT FLASHES

of temperatures over 100° on the day of the wedding.

There was a time when I believed that because of the anxiety I felt during perimenopause, I might never even be able to attend my son's wedding. A number of months earlier, I could not even handle going out to dinner without being panic-stricken, but I was able to fly four thousand miles to be with my son on his special day with no problem. Anxiety! Now that's another story.

HOW TO SURVIVE MENOPAUSE WITHOUT GOING CRAZY

FROM MILD ANXIETY TO FULL-FLEDGED PANIC ATTACKS

CHAPTER 3

FROM MILD ANXIETY TO FULL-FLEDGED PANIC ATTACKS

Palpitations were not new to 50-year-old Sandy. In fact, she had experienced them on and off for years. She had learned to live with them after being diagnosed with a prolapsed valve, often associated with heart palpitations and after an unsuccessful treatment trial of Inderal. Relaxation technique usually helped and the palpitations proved to be nothing more than an inconvenience. Until one afternoon while making the usual short drive from work to her home. Sandy's mother, with whom she had had a close and loving relationship, had died a couple of years earlier, and as she drove past the house where her mother had lived, she was literally struck by a devastating episode of panic. She could not breathe. Her heart was pounding so loudly and so quickly that she felt she was going to pass out and indeed, believes she may have "blacked out" for a little while. She was almost totally immobilized by this panic attack, but did manage to pull her car off to the side of the road until the episode subsided.

This traumatic occurrence followed by a couple of less severe ones when she was behind the wheel led Sandy to be frightened by the thought of driving alone. However, she fought this phobic reaction to the panic attack and forced herself to make the daily drive to and from town.

HOW TO SURVIVE MENOPAUSE
WITHOUT GOING CRAZY

Then, Sandy experienced another panic attack, once again being taken totally by surprise at both the severity and nature of the occurrence. Sandy, who along with her husband of 29 years, has spent more time on the water than on land was in her cabin getting ready for a cruise to Cozumal. Once again, she was overcome by overwhelming feelings of anxiety that made her feel if she did not flee the ship immediately, she would surely die. Instead, she made herself relax until her rapidly beating heart slowed and the feelings of panic eased.

Why all of a sudden did Sandy begin experiencing anxiety attacks and what does all of this have to do with menopause? After all, an estimated 12 million people, maybe more, experience some sort of panic attack from time to time, and although most are women, this condition is certainly not limited to menopausal women. Is anxiety really related to menopause since not all menopausal women complain of this symptom?

As Vilet and Davis point out, most symptoms of depression and anxiety do show up in women during their mid 30's and 40's and research suggests "there is a previously unrecognized connection between declining hormone levels in this age group of females and the high incidence of depression and anxiety." These authors go on to discuss this relationship at length. They differentiate between those major anxiety disorders that often need psychiatric intervention and those associated with perimenopause. They believe that symptoms of anxiety during menopause are less severe and are directly related to the menstrual cycle of those women in perimenopause still experiencing menses, even though periods may be irregular. They have found anxiety usually occurs 3-5 days prior to one's menstrual period when estrogen levels are low and progesterone levels are higher.

Of course, other factors may be involved in the appearance and increased incidence of anxiety and panic attacks during perimenopause. We now know that estrogen and progesterone affect endorphins, brain chemicals that enhance our sense of well-being and may have a calming effect during anxiety states. Increased estrogen levels are definitely related

FROM MILD ANXIETY TO FULL-FLEDGED PANIC ATTACKS

to increased endorphin levels. Also, as discussed earlier, an increased adrenalin output during hot flashes may also be responsible for varying levels of anxiety.

* * * *

I begin having occasional anxiety attacks a year or so before I was even aware I was menopausal. I didn't know what was happening to me at first. Because I come from a family of diabetics, I thought the feelings of dizziness and lightheadedness that I felt at times might indicate a problem with my blood sugar. Also, I would have the quick little flash of anxiety before my face turned red, but this happened only once or twice, so I didn't even know that I was "hot flashing" at first.

After my physician ruled out diabetes and ruled in perimenopause, I began taking Premarin and Provera. The periodic episodes of anxiety continued, however, almost always occurring in the late afternoon or early evening. I had no idea why this was happening to me. What could be causing the increased number of anxiety attacks? Were they brought on by the hot flashes, by something I was eating (they happened mostly around the evening meal), by stress, by the Provera I was taking? Could it be the estrogen pill I was taking in the morning was out of my system by late afternoon?

My journal entries reflect my frustration at determining what was causing these increased incidences of panic:

Wednesday, Oct. 23, 5p.m.
Hard to describe what I am feeling. No appetite, a little weak. No stomach problems. Fairly anxious with a wave of anxiety- type feeling. Very hypersensitive to cooking smells when I walked at 6p.m.

Food: Egg at breakfast with bagel. Tuna salad with tomato at lunch. Peanuts. Herbal tea. Forced self to eat peanut butter toast at dinner.

Emotional/Stress: Mike gone. Day before first tutoring session for literacy program.

HOW TO SURVIVE MENOPAUSE
WITHOUT GOING CRAZY

Hormones: 23'rd day of estrogen. 8th day of Provera. Period should begin 26th.

Other: Very warm day. In the 90's.

Action: Ate peanut butter toast, milk. Took a walk. Tried to refocus. Said my prayers. Fair results. Did not have to take an anti-anxiety pill.

Friday, Nov. 2, 7:00 p.m.
Definite hot flash, but only a little anxious. Flash lasted a couple of minutes. Stomach upset. Took several deep breaths.

Food: Bagel. Turkey on French at lunch. Dinner out at about 6:30 consisted of fried clams, shrimp, Sprite.

Emotional/Stress: At very noisy Spurs game.

Hormones: First day of estrogen after normal 7 day period.

Other: Very loud game. Cool weather, but felt warm in the arena.

Action: Took deep breaths. Did not need anti-anxiety meds.

Saturday, Nov. 9, 4:30 p.m.
Hot flash? Only brief wave of heat. Stomach very upset. A little free-floating anxiety.

Food: Cereal, Chicken noodle soup and shrimp with hot sauce at 3:30 p.m.

FROM MILD ANXIETY TO FULL-FLEDGED PANIC ATTACKS

Emotional/Stress: Lack of sleep for past 3 days due to sinusitis and taking antihistamines, antibiotic, and cortisone nasal spray as well as aspirin.

Hormonal: 9th day of estrogen

Other: Possibly overheated from wearing heavy warm-ups. Stomach upset from aspirin and perhaps the antibiotic.

Action: Moved around and tried to refocus. Wrote in this journal. No antianxiety drug taken. Listened to relaxation tape instead.

Saturday, Dec. 7, 10:30 p.m.
Left Christmas party early. One hot flash after another with much anxiety, hypersensitivity to smells, lack of appetite. Some nausea and diarrhea, also.

Food: Bagel, juice, chicken salad at lunch. Tangerine and milk about 5 p.m. One glass of wine at 7 p.m. Unable to eat dinner.

Emotional/Stress: Very warm at the party. Band was extremely loud. Shrimp were strong-smelling. General stress I always experience during the holidays.

Other: Could not remove very heavy and hot dress with sequins and room remained hot and stuffy.

Action: Took Atarax 10 mg. and pepto-bismal, but it didn't help. Came home early and after I cooled down and calmed down, I felt better.

What I learned from the journal is when I was stressed out or hot or did

HOW TO SURVIVE MENOPAUSE
WITHOUT GOING CRAZY

anything to bring on a hot flash, chances are I was also going to experience anxiety on some level. I also learned the episodes of anxiety occurred only in the late afternoon or early evening, never during the day. I asked my gynecologist if the Premarin pill could be "wearing off" by the end of the day, but he said he did not believe this was happening. However, Dr. Raymond Burnett in *Menopause: All Your Questions Answered* points out the fact that some women do indeed "metabolize or excrete" oral estrogen more rapidly than others. Another factor that could have contributed to the early evening hot flashes and consequent anxiety attacks is discussed by Dr. Sadja Greenwood in *Menopause Naturally: Preparing for the Second Half of Life*. She found that hot flashes occur more frequently between 6 and 9 p.m.

    I discovered another important contributing factor to the increased number and severity of anxiety attacks. Very often they occurred during the last couple of days of Provera treatment and especially during the period when I had no hormones in my body. I had experienced only mild PMS prior to perimenopause, so what was happening to me now was very similar, but much worse. I have learned since that many women have PMS-type problems when taking Provera. But, I believed and still do believe it is absolutely necessary to continue it as an adjunct to the estrogen therapy. We need it to prevent the dreaded, but rare endometrial cancer I had been repeatedly cautioned about before beginning HRT.

    As I told you in the introduction to this book and as my journal reflected, the anxiety, somewhat mild at first, became progressively worse, and I decided I needed to do something about it. After that fiasco with the female psychiatrist, and after learning that my estrogen level was still pretty low, my gynecologist and I decided to try the estrogen patch instead of the more familiar Premarin tablet. Switching to the patch helped tremendously, because I could now get a slow, but steady, uninterrupted amount of estrogen 24 hours a day. I had fewer hot flashes which meant less anxiety. But during times of stress especially, I continued to have pretty severe panic attacks. I learned to wear two .05 mg. patches during these periods.

FROM MILD ANXIETY TO FULL-FLEDGED PANIC ATTACKS

When I knew I was going to be involved in something especially stressful, like my son's wedding or when I had to deal with my special friend's death from breast cancer, I took Atarax (a mild antianxiety medication) for very brief periods of time. I don't like taking medication unless absolutely necessary, so I was feeling pretty hopeless during this time about my chances of returning to normal. Anyway, despite these two major interventions, I still worried that I would become phobic if I did not get a handle on the anxiety. I read everything I could get my hands on about anxiety, panic attacks and phobia. I found one book that was literally a life saver for me. *The Panic Attack Recovery Book* by Shirley Swede and Seymour Sheppard Jaffe, M.D. really did help me deal with my anxiety. In fact, from the moment they acknowledged that "many normal people experience some degree of panic from time to time" and that it might occur during a "period of hormonal change such as the onset of puberty or menopause," I knew they had something to contribute in the way of relief from the symptoms. They offer a seven part program that consists of diet, relaxation, exercise, the right attitude, imaging, social support, and spiritual values. Since the program is consistent with other programs for menopausal women, it will be discussed further in Chapter 12.

It was encouraging to learn that I was on the right track in terms of the steps I had already taken to survive this horrible consequence of menopause. I walked and did aerobics daily. I had stopped smoking and had cut out caffeine, fats and salt from my diet. I took a multivitamin along with calcium daily. I added B Complex after reading the book. I also used relaxation techniques when I felt particularly stressed out. The book also provided new facts about attitude and mental approach to conquering anxiety attacks. This information was the most helpful to me.

Anyway, once I became aware that I was not crazy, that many women developed anxiety attacks during perimenopause, I was on my way to recovery. This was something I could learn to deal with until I passed to the other side of menopause. I also learned that although I may have setbacks when I am particularly stressed, I will not become phobic. And

HOW TO SURVIVE MENOPAUSE
WITHOUT GOING CRAZY

if I do, I'll be able to handle that, too.

I mentioned taking Atarax periodically. It is actually an antihistamine that works as an antianxiety drug. It's been around for years and years and has very few side effects. Besides Xanax that the psychiatrist prescribed for me (which I decided not to try), other anti-anxiety agents are often prescribed. Ativan, Serax, Valium, Librium, Klonipin, and Buspar are some of the better-known ones. As I said earlier, I am not too fond of taking medication and only do so after becoming well-informed about what I'm putting into my body. You should do the same. After trying all the non-drug treatments for menopausal associated anxiety, if you decide to go the medication route, be sure your doctor tells you all possible side effects, if the drug is addicting, how much and how long you should take the drug, and how the drug will make you feel.

Acknowledging that feelings of anxiety and panic may very well be related to menopause is the first step in heading off possible devastating effects of this symptom. Once you accept this basic fact, you can move on to the other steps mentioned in this chapter that have worked for me and many others. It is so great to once again feel excited rather than anxious about someone, some thing or some event.

DEPRESSION: TEARFULNESS, MOOD SWINGS, JUST PLAIN BLAHS

CHAPTER 4

DEPRESSION: TEARFULNESS, MOOD SWINGS, JUST PLAIN BLAHS

Like many menopausal women, 48-year-old Kathy is still not sure the severe bouts of depression that have caused her to feel suicidal at times are even related to the change. She is in the perimenopausal stage of life, still having menstrual periods. The mood swings, tearfulness, and sadness usually occur the week before her menses begins. Kathy often has trouble sleeping and is irritable and tired every day. She also has problems with concentration and is very forgetful. Kathy's depression was serious enough for her to seek professional help. Although she is still "fearful and anxious" at times, with the help of antidepressant medication, she is beginning to sleep better. She also reports she is starting to "feel the depression lifting."

A friend of mine thought I should name this book, *The Pause That Depresses*. I laughed at this suggestion because although I had every other strange and awful thing it was possible to have during menopause, I was not depressed. At least I didn't think I was at the time. Of course, I could very well have been too depressed to know I was depressed. But, because I didn't feel depressed, I didn't think it was a major problem for other women either.

However, as I began my research for this book, I learned differently. We've already discussed the fact that in the past menopausal women were even hospitalized for depression or melancholia as it was called. Yet,

HOW TO SURVIVE MENOPAUSE WITHOUT GOING CRAZY

almost every modern-day scientific publication states with authority that women are not any more depressed because of menopause than usual. This blanket statement from the medical profession in particular makes a lot of us women angry as was the case with Marcie when she received the brochure from her local hospital.

Many other authorities on menopause have supported this outright denial of increased incidents of depression during menopause despite the lack of conclusive evidence and shortage of research studies on the subject. The following excerpt from a fairly recent book is typical of this point of view:

> *"Modern medicine concedes that there is no clear-cut cause and effect relationship between menopause and depression."*
> Gretchen Henkel, Making the Estrogen Decision, 1992

Ms. Henkel's voice is just one of many that reports no relationship between menopause and depression. Recently, I heard Dr. Judith Reichman discussing menopause on public TV. She also was emphatic in her assertion that there is no increase in psychiatric illness during menopause. Yet, if we look to other authorities on the subject of menopause and psychiatric illness, especially depression, about half will take the exact opposite view.

In Dr. Burnett's book, for example, he shows depression as 3'rd at 78% in his list of symptoms of menopause and the frequency of occurrence. Another well-known author, Lila Nachttigall, M.D., who writes about the emotional component of menopause in her book, *Estrogen: The Facts Can Change Your Life*, also lists depression among the signs of menopause.

We women don't like to think of menopause itself as a disease. In fact, some of us were upset because PMS was listed in the revised DSM III, the diagnostic manual that defines psychiatric illness for mental health professionals. It is understandable that we do not wish to be thought of as

DEPRESSION: TEARFULNESS, MOOD SWINGS, JUST PLAIN BLAHS

incapacitated in any way because of our hormones, or by the mere fact that we are females. And while I agree with this philosophy, I also believe we should not be afraid to admit our problems and to seek help for them when necessary. Menopause is a stage of life, not a disease. Although, I use the word, *symptom*, many times in describing what happens to us during menopause, I do not use the word in the clinical sense. I am merely describing the signs of menopause. But, I also use the word, *problem*, a great deal. When a sign or symptom becomes a problem that makes it difficult for us to function or even to achieve a good quality of life, then it may be time to seek professional help.

Anxiety, as I found out, is one of those problems that may cause one to start looking for a mental health professional. Depression is another. Whether or not Kathy's depression is connected to her menopause is not the most important consideration. What matters is that when she realized she had a potentially incapacitating problem, she sought help for it. However, it might have been helpful, perhaps even a relief for Kathy to know her depression was possibly related to menopause, if not caused by the fluctuation in hormones, then at least exacerbated by it.

In reviewing the literature, I found that most authors do deal with the issue of depression and menopause to some degree. As I said, about 50% deny there is any connection at all between the two. The other 50% are quick to demonstrate a definite link between menopause and depression.

So who should we believe? Or does it even matter that we accept either of these two opposing opinions? One of the major problems seems to be that many authors choose to define depression differently. We need to understand the definitions, especially the difference between mild, menopausal blues and severe, clinical depression.

Gail Sheehy is one of the authors who does try to clarify the issue by making the distinction. In *The Silent Passage: Menopause*, she says, "Women low in estrogen often have feelings of malaise, as opposed to suffering from the DSM-III criteria of depression as disease..." She goes on to discuss the *temporary* nature of the "blues" women experience

HOW TO SURVIVE MENOPAUSE
WITHOUT GOING CRAZY

during perimenopause.

In the scientific article by Vliet, et. al. mentioned in Chapter 1, the authors list the symptoms for major or clinical depression. They point out that at least five of the following symptoms need to be present for at least 2 weeks, "despite pleasant life event":

1. Mood changes such as irritability, feeling sad or discouraged. Loss of interest in usual activities. Social withdrawal.

2. Increased or decreased appetite. Weight gain or loss. Too much or too little sleep. Loss of interest in sex. Fatigue.

3. Body movements and/or speech becomes slower. Feeling of restlessness or being "keyed up."

4. Diminished memory, decreased concentration, feelings of worthlessness, guilt. Thoughts of suicide, or preoccupation with death.

It's interesting that so many of these signs of major depression are also discussed in this book as signs of menopause. No wonder the authorities can't agree on the relationship between depression and menopause. You need to understand, however, that although irritability and fatigue, for example, might be signs of depression, they might also be signs of menopause caused by lack of sleep, in turn, caused by nighttime hot flashes, brought on by estrogen deprivation. In other words, irritability and fatigue may be symptoms of menopause rather than depression, or both. And, the same goes for memory and concentration problems. These signs, like irritability and fatigue, are almost always present during menopause and may be due to various other causes besides depression as proposed in the following chapters.

However, if you are feeling unusually sad, and also have some of the other symptoms mentioned above, particularly, sustained or prolonged feelings of hopelessness, slowed body movements and speech, sleeping all the time, and thoughts of suicide, you should not hesitate to seek medical attention as soon as possible. If, on the other hand, you find yourself a little blue or moody at times, chances are these feelings will go away without medical intervention.

DEPRESSION: TEARFULNESS, MOOD SWINGS, JUST PLAIN BLAHS

I told you in the introduction to this book how despite not feeling depressed, I cried periodically for the most ridiculous of reasons. I shed tears of joy and sorrow. Sometimes the tears flowed for no apparent reason at all. No one seems to know what causes these emotional overflow of tears, but so many menopausal women report them, you are certainly not alone. I associated my tears with my ever-changing and unpredictable moods in general during perimenopause.

* * * *

Marilyn, whose menopausal symptoms began around age 49 or 50, actually experienced very few of the problems usually associated with the change. Except for overwhelming feelings of depression that, like Kathy's, were serious enough for her to seek medical attention. Marilyn is doing much better now and recently wrote about her experiences on my questionnaire: "During the course of menopause, and in hindsight, I recognize that many symptoms I thought could be attributed to the breakup of my marriage might have been influenced by hormonal changes. In fact, lots of things such as forgetfulness, lack of concentration, I have attributed to aging process, not menopause."

Marilyn brings up an interesting point. Was her depression related exclusively to the breakup of her long-lasting marriage? What role, if any, did menopause play in what happened to her? So many authorities today are eager to blame several possible life changes we women undergo in our late 40's and early 50's for any mental health problems we may have during menopause. Divorce, the empty-nest syndrome, changes in job status, fear of aging and death are just a few of the culprits often mentioned as causing the depression and other psychological problems some of us have during this time.

Is there some truth to theory that life changes are responsible for the emotional upheaval we sometimes experience during menopause? I remember how I vehemently denied to the female psychiatrist that my anxiety was in any way caused by the fact that I was undergoing stressful

HOW TO SURVIVE MENOPAUSE
WITHOUT GOING CRAZY

changes in my life. "On the contrary," I explained to her, "I am certainly not experiencing the so-called empty-nest syndrome." In fact, at the time of this discussion, my children had been on their own for a number of years, and both were doing exceptionally well. Although some of us will never regret it when the teenage years come to an end, seeing our children reach adulthood is really special. To know that we've done a good job bringing them up, or at least the best job that we knew how to do, thus assuring them a happy and successful place in society. Because of how we raised them and sometimes miraculously, despite how we raised them. I mean, a part of us is always sad when our babies grow up and leave home. But, this life event is not usually the cause for major depression.

And yes, also around this time some of our marriages, like Marilyn's, do end in divorce. But Marilyn had been preparing for the separation from her husband for a number of years. And she sought the divorce only after her children had grown as she had been planning to do for a long time. She and her ex-husband have remained close friends. Still, it doesn't matter if the separation from your spouse or loved one is through divorce or death, it is still a loss and you can expect to grieve for a period of time. Marilyn knew she was going to mourn the end of her marriage despite being prepared for it. She did not, however, expect the serious depression that followed. Of course, I imagine if her husband had left her for a young chick-a-dee with big bazoons as some "menopausal men" are inclined to do, that might have been a whole different story.

Which brings us to another life change that may or may not cause us to feel somewhat depressed. The aging process. If you remember, originally Marilyn believed the aging process rather than menopause was responsible for some of her problems such as forgetfulness and lack of concentration. It is doubtful that aging alone is responsible for those two symptoms as you will see in the following chapters. However, the aging process is another loss for all of us, the loss of our youth.

There comes a time when we look in the mirror, and we see the tell-tale lines and sagging begin to appear. And, we do feel sad about our lost

DEPRESSION: TEARFULNESS, MOOD SWINGS, JUST PLAIN BLAHS

youthfulness. Once again, though, we are not so depressed about these unwelcome changes that we need to seek medical attention. I have found that our initial unhappiness at the discovery that we are getting older is usually replaced by an inner call to action. Some of us get plastic surgery; others less inclined to suffer physical pain try new make-up, different hairstyles, take up aerobics or find a personal trainer. We go on diets, stop smoking to halt further wrinkling. I believe it is not the getting older so much that bothers us, but the physical manifestations of that process. So, in the end, either we accept the changes that come along with aging, or like most of us, we use the many tools available to us today to slow the face of aging, if not the process itself.

Most traumatic life events can cause temporary bouts of major depressive episodes, but temporary is the key. I realize that some of us who have devoted our whole lives to our children may indeed experience the empty-nest syndrome. And some of us whose husbands leave us through mutual (or otherwise) divorce or through death will certainly be saddened by the loss. And, those of us who are asked to take an early retirement from a job that may have fulfilled us for years are definitely going to grieve for the emptiness we now feel. But, the depression we experience because of events, the way we react to sad events in our lives is different than the debilitating, clinical or major depression that occurs "despite pleasant life events." And, it helps to know, although we may not believe it, especially during these devastating periods of our lives, time will indeed help to heal in the case of depression due to loss.

The years surrounding menopause, then, can certainly be a time of life-altering social change. These life changes can and do affect our emotional stability. But don't forget that you are also going through tremendous hormonal changes which can also affect your mental health especially during perimenopause. Neither of these two forces, however, should cause serious clinical depression. They may make your depression worse if you're already depressed. And whether your depression is related to hormonal or social change or both, it is usually of a temporary nature. Once

HOW TO SURVIVE MENOPAUSE
WITHOUT GOING CRAZY

again, you need to decide if your depression is typical menopausal blues. Or serious depression caused by a change in your life and exacerbated by hormonal change. Or major depression despite good things happening in your life and also helped on by hormonal imbalance. The last two may indicate it's time to look for professional help even if the depression is temporary.

So, what can you do about depression. First, of all the "blahs." If the mild menopausal depression or malaise you experience during menopause is caused by a hormonal imbalance, then estrogen supplementation should help. Many authors speak of the so-called mood enhancement effect of hormone replacement. Wulf Utian, M.D., Ph.D. was one of the first to report a relationship between estrogen replacement and an enhanced feeling of well-being. He makes no claim that estrogen acts as an antidepressant, but believes it does help us feel better mood-wise. He calls estrogen's action, a "mental tonic effect." It's important to note here that although estrogen is believed by many to improve mood, the progestin given along with estrogen in hormone replacement therapy has been known to cause depression in some women. We need to weigh the benefits of taking progestin against the degree of depression we may feel for a few days during the month. We'll discuss progestin further in Chapter 12.

Besides estrogen replacement to help cure the blues, exercise is probably the most widely recommended method by professionals. It is a well-know fact that exercise increases the serotonin levels in the brain, causing the so-called runner's high. Before you begin an exercise program, consult your physician or an exercise physiologist to help you decide what's right for you. Then choose something that's fun for you. I took up biking. But, I live in a hilly area and was always afraid I was going to crack my head open as I sped downhill at 70 miles an hour, slightly out of control. Walking is perhaps the best way to start. I usually walk a couple of miles a day. I also do aerobics with Denise on TV. Although she does too much step aerobics for my taste, she has an excellent weight lifting program that I feel helps prevent osteoporosis. Weight bearing exercise is recommended

DEPRESSION: TEARFULNESS, MOOD SWINGS, JUST PLAIN BLAHS

along with estrogen and calcium supplements for women at high risk for developing this dreaded bone disease.

So, if you have the menopausal blues, both estrogen replacement and an exercise program should help. What else can you do to get through this phase with a minimum of trauma. Try some of the following suggestions:

1. Eat healthy. Stay off sugars, caffeine, and alcohol for a more balanced, stable mood. Too much of any of these can cause some real fluctuations in highs and lows.

2. Some nutritionists recommend B Vitamin supplements, especially Vitamin B6. Talk with your doctor or pharmacist about how much to take, since an over-dosage can be toxic. I take 50 mg. of a time-released B Complex.

3. Do some of the personal care things mentioned above. Take care of your hair and skin. Lose weight. Stop smoking. Buy new clothes.

4. If you don't have a job, and you no longer need to devote as much time to your family, find some purpose in life to keep you happy and busy. Join clubs, go back to school, find a new job or change careers. Take up writing, painting, sewing. Whatever. Just decide that the second half of your life has just begun. Then be determined to make it better, more fulfilling than the first half.

If you determine that your depression is serious and that you are truly having trouble coping with everyday life, then it is probably time to consult a professional. Although a psychologist, social worker, or other licensed mental health worker may be equally qualified to treat you, only a psychiatrist can prescribe anti-depressant medication. The others can refer you to a psychiatrist for just that purpose. There are many good anti-depressant drugs around today, the most popular, of course, is Prozac, given frequently now to help women with PMS.

One of the most important factors in determining who to see may be how well-informed that therapist is on the matter of menopause. If the psychotherapist you have chosen immediately dismisses the relationship between menopause and depression and blames it all on life changes, he or

HOW TO SURVIVE MENOPAUSE
WITHOUT GOING CRAZY

she is not going to be much help to you. Look for a modern, well-informed therapist who can discuss all options for you. Your depression may not be caused by hormone deprivation or fluctuation, but it can certainly be exacerbated by it. Just going through the numerous physical and gynecological changes, as well as the emotional and social changes can cause or at least intensify a depressive episode. A good psychotherapist will understand this and be able to act on it.

So much is still unknown about how major depression is affected by menopause or how menopause affects it. But, we do know how to treat serious depression if it occurs. It's up to you to seek that help if you need it. Menopausal blues on the other hand is just one more bane of the change that you need to get through the best you can. I haven't mentioned a support group, but if you've tried all of the other suggestions, and you still fell blah a lot of the time, you might want to gather a few of your menopausal friends for meetings on a regular basis. Misery really does love company in the case of menopause. I always felt so much better knowing some of the women I loved and cared about were just as miserable as I was.

INSOMNIA & OTHER SLEEP DISTURBANCES

CHAPTER 5

INSOMNIA & OTHER SLEEP DISTURBANCES

It's 2:45 a.m. and I'm wide awake again. I don't know what has awakened me. In the past, I have been awakened by hot flashes, and even by night sweats. A few times I remember being jerked awake by nightmares. But, most of the time I just find myself awake at 3 o'clock in the morning. It's the most awful feeling. Knowing that if I don't get back to sleep, I'm going to feel worthless all day. Yet, the harder I try, the more difficult it is. So, I get up and I read, or I watch TV or I write. Whatever. But, I'd rather be asleep.

I wrote this in the middle of the night, long before my gynecologist and I found the correct dosage of estrogen to stop the hot flashes. Sleep problems have plagued me from the very beginning of my menopausal journey.

Sleeplessness is a major menopausal problem. Almost every woman I contacted experienced it. The causes are various, but the major reason women experience disturbed sleep is because they are having hot flashes. They awaken to find themselves throwing the covers off only to find themselves cold just a few minutes later and pulling them back up. Or they may awaken because their nightclothes are literally drenched with perspiration. They get up to change them and find they cannot get back to sleep. Some women are awakened by nightmares that are reportedly more frequent during menopause. And quite a few women are awakened by heart palpitations and in some cases, panic attacks.

HOW TO SURVIVE MENOPAUSE WITHOUT GOING CRAZY

* * * *

63-year-old Ella began having menopausal symptoms at age 40 and she vividly remembers the very first time she was abruptly awakened in the middle of the night by a terrifying panic attack. Ella continued to have these "spells" as she called her frequent episodes of palpitations and nervousness for several years. She suffered sleep problems nightly despite HRT. Ella does not attribute her sleep disturbance to hot flashes which she has never experienced at all. She firmly believes her sleeplessness is related to the panic attacks which "always occurred during the night."

* * * *

Louise, like Ella, also awakens abruptly during the night. Louise is a youthful looking 48-year-old grandmother who is currently experiencing several of the symptoms associated with the emotional component of perimenopause. "I have learned to live with all these symptoms," she writes. "The only time I find it rough is at night when I wake up fearful. This seems to happen once every couple of months. It is a horrible feeling and I am afraid to go back to sleep once I calm myself down, afraid it is going to happen again . . ."

* * * *

Brenda is an active 54-year-old who has not allowed some pretty significant symptoms of menopause that she began experiencing around the age of 50 slow her down. Her major discomfort was from "wakefulness and hot flashes." Brenda dealt with her sleep problems as she deals with everything else in her life. With a positive attitude and eternal optimism. She says of her insomnia: "I've never been a great sleeper. My internist gave me a mild dose of Elavil ...about a year ago and now I sleep like a baby! I still get night sweats occasionally - in the beginning, it was very frequent."

Ella, Louise, Brenda and I all experienced sleep problems associated with menopause, but for each of us it seems a different precipitating factor was involved. Ella was awakened by panic attacks, Louise by unnamed

INSOMNIA & OTHER SLEEP DISTURBANCES

fearfulness, Brenda by night sweats and I by undetermined reasons that are mostly associated with hot flashes since I always feel warm when I awaken early in the morning. For me, fewer hot flashes means better sleep.

Several theories concerning the reasons for sleep disturbance in menopausal women have been proposed. The most common one, of course, is the occurrence of hot flashes caused by a drop in estrogen levels. Sleep studies have shown that nighttime hot flashes do indeed cause women to awaken in the middle of the night.

One writer, Lila Nachtigall, M.D., in *Estrogen: The Facts Can Change Your Life* says the lack of sleep some menopausal women experience may not be due exclusively to hot flashes as the majority of experts maintain. She believes the insomnia "is also caused by changes in sleep pattern and brain waves from the same hypothalamic disturbances that result in hot flashes and an overstimulated central nervous system." Dr. Nachtigall goes on to describe a common nocturnal pattern that many menopausal women experience and that is awakening in the early morning with the inability to go back to sleep.

Some medical authorities believe sleeplessness may also be caused by depression. As we have discussed in Chapter 4, many women experience depression during the menopause transition. It seems no one really knows if depression does indeed cause sleeplessness or if sleeplessness causes depression as others have proposed.

We do know that chronic lack of sleep can cause some real emotional disturbances, and in menopausal women, is probably the major cause of irritability, fatigue, moodiness, problems with concentration, tenseness. You name it. If we are going to feel good both mentally and physically we need to get adequate sleep. And sleep deprivation can cause some serious problems.

So, even if we don't know for sure what is causing the sleep disturbance, we do know we will have to do something about it sooner or later. What to do about sleeplessness is a different matter. If you are being awakened by hot flashes and night sweats as are most menopausal women,

HOW TO SURVIVE MENOPAUSE
WITHOUT GOING CRAZY

then the solution to the problem is simple. Get rid of the hot flashes. We discussed ways to deal with this most common complaint in Chapter 2.

There are also ways to deal with insomnia that sleep experts recommend despite the cause of sleeplessness. I have found most of these extremely helpful.

1. Always go to bed at the same time and always awaken at the same time.

2. If you can't get to sleep, don't just lay there and toss and turn for hours. Get up after 10 to 20 minutes and do something that is relaxing for you.

3. If you awaken in the middle of the night or in the early morning hours and cannot get back to sleep, do the same thing, get out of bed and do something.

4. Exercise may help, but always exercise in the late afternoon or early in the evening so you'll have time to relax before retiring for the evening.

5. Take a warm bath to totally relax your muscles. Make sure the water is not too hot since this is one way to invite a hot flash.

6. Have a snack before going to bed. Stay away from caffeine and alcohol. Sugar before bedtime is also taboo. Instead, carbohydrates are usually always recommended. Warm milk is also a good choice. I always like to combine a little piece of cheese, a slice of apple and glass of milk. An old wives tale perhaps started me on this combination, but it works for me. Do whatever works for you.

7. Take some quiet time and do whatever relaxes you. A favorite tape perhaps, soothing music, a relaxation exercise, meditation, and/or prayer.

8. The latest recommendation by sleep scientists is not to use the bedroom for extracurricular activity. However, even at the height of my own sleep problems, I always fell right asleep during Jay Leno's dialogue. Sorry, Jay.

9. It is extremely important for menopausal women that the bedroom be cool. So turn on the air-conditioner, the fan or open the window if necessary. Do not try to sleep in a hot, stuffy room.

INSOMNIA & OTHER SLEEP DISTURBANCES

10. Many menopausal women experience frequency of urination, so try to avoid drinking a lot of liquids right before you go to bed.

11. Get up at the same time every morning even if you don't feel you got enough sleep the night before and never take naps in the afternoon. In other words, develop your own sleep schedule.

12. I haven't found anyone who recommends over the counter sleeping pills. In fact, their use is almost always discouraged. However, if you have tried everything and nothing works, your physician may prescribe a sleeping pill for temporary relief. The key word here is *temporary*. We've all heard about the problems associated with the popular sleeping pill, Halcion, a prescription drug.

The most common sleep problem reported by menopausal women is unsound sleep. We may get to sleep with no problem, but we awaken frequently during the night or in the early morning hours as Dr. Nachtigall reported. And, as I can well verify. Some of the latest research findings on sleep disturbance show a definite relationship between body temperature and sleep problems. The normal person's temperature goes down at night. Insomniacs don't cool down as much at night, so they experience fragmented or broken sleep. We can easily see then, another connection between unsound sleep and the menopausal woman who is having hot flashes and night sweats. So once again, getting rid of the hot flashes is one major step toward better sleep.

Finally, it is important to remember that we all need different amounts of sleep. Our bodies will let us know if we're not getting enough. If you awaken after only four or five hours feeling refreshed and energetic, you probably don't need more than that. If on the other hand, you feel rotten, irritable and sleepy, try some of the remedies mentioned above. I felt great after estrogen therapy relieved my hot flashes enough for me to get two or three uninterrupted nights of sleep in a row. You will, too.

If you cannot or choose not to take estrogen, try some of the other suggestions listed above. If you still can find no relief for your sleep problems, you might want to contact the National Sleep Foundation at

HOW TO SURVIVE MENOPAUSE
WITHOUT GOING CRAZY

(310)288-0466 or write them at 122 S. Robertson Blvd., Los Angeles, CA 90048. Help is available.

IMPATIENCE: ONLY ONE SIGN OF IRRITABILITY

CHAPTER 6

IMPATIENCE: ONLY ONE SIGN OF IRRITABILITY

Marcie's oldest daughter, Sharon, was a college freshman when she first discovered the danger of confronting a irritable menopausal woman. Sharon was home for the holidays and was in the bathroom putting away freshly laundered towels when Marcie walked in and began complaining about having a hot flash. "I don't know what you're whining about," Sharon joked. "It must be wonderful not to be bothered by those messy monthly periods." Sharon was totally unprepared for the bitter retort that practically spewed from her mother in about two seconds. "You have no idea what I'm going through. I have to deal with hot flashes, dryness, incontinence, anxiety, headaches, ..." Without taking a breath, Marcie went on to list another five or so other scourges of menopause, and poor Sharon never dared to mention the advantages of menopause to her mother again.

Marcie went on to tell her daughter that until she actually experienced menopause one day, she could never even imagine what it's like. When describing this scene to me, Sharon said of the changes her Mom and other menopausal women experience in terms of irritability, "It's as if all the sacrifices are over. They are no longer willing to take the smallest piece of the cake."

My 24-year-old daughter, Allison and I were talking about this Jekyll and Hyde aspect of menopause. "We become mean," I told Allison. "It's

HOW TO SURVIVE MENOPAUSE
WITHOUT GOING CRAZY

like we have this sudden need to take care of ourselves, because no one else is going to take care of us." My husband, who had made his share of sacrifices for me during the really rough times of my menopause, perked up at these words. "We begin asserting ourselves, maybe for the first time," I continued. "We'll do anything to make ourselves feel better."

Allison tried to compare the irritability we experience at the time of menopause to the PMS symptoms she experiences monthly. And, there are lots of similarities. We can feel so tense that the expression, "I feel like jumping out of my skin" becomes real for us. The mother/child, wife/husband relationship can become very strained at this time. One fellow in my writer's group said his mother, a normally placid lady, was impatient and irritable for 10 years. They had no idea until recently when people began talking about menopause, that that's what was happening to her.

I remember seeing an episode of *All In The Family* years ago when Edith Bunker went through the "change." The normally sweet-mannered, always pleasant Edith suddenly became irritable, moody and pretty bitchy. Archie and Gloria and Mike were at a complete loss as to how to deal with this disagreeable stranger in their lives. It was a very funny show. But, this often sudden aggressiveness that sometimes appears during menopause is not a laughing matter. Our behavior can become very threatening to our loved ones. A friend of mine jokingly told me that she became so irritated with her husband at times, she really felt like killing him. Although, she tried to make light of the matter, I knew she was really bothered by her lack of intolerance for her husband's small annoyances that had been going on for years. Like Archie, our husbands are totally unprepared for the changes we go through.

Even more precarious is the mother/child, especially the mother/daughter relationship. Women usually experience menopause around the time their children leave home for college or their first jobs. The children are just beginning their own lives as adults. In recent years, however, our children have begun to leave the nest later or are returning for financial reasons. They are getting a closer look at this phenomenon called

IMPATIENCE: ONLY ONE SIGN OF IRRITABILITY

menopause that their Mom's are in the clutches of. Said one young and very concerned 22-year-old, "I'm really worried about my mother. She's having such a "bad" menopause. She's just not herself." Young women want to understand what's happening to their mothers because they know that they'll be going through this stage of life themselves someday. They want to know the truth about menopause so they can move through the phase with less fright. They know if they are better prepared and better informed, the transition will be a lot easier for them. At least, better than it is for their mothers, the women of my generation, many of whom are entering this significant time of their lives almost blind.

* * * *

I have always been an assertive person. I didn't become really aggressive, however, til I became menopausal. During one week at the height of my newly found passion for affirming my rights, needs, and desires rather dramatically, I:

    a. Wrote to a food company and complained that their graham crackers tasted "sinfully bad."

    b. Called the customer service manager of a local department store to insist that he honor a telephone agreement to ship my order before Christmas. I had received a letter stating it would be 6 to 8 weeks after initially being told it would arrive in a couple of weeks. After shaming him by saying his store really didn't know how to do business, I threatened never to shop there again.

    c. Nastily told a carpet salesperson, who was pressuring us to purchase a carpet immediately because it would "no longer be on sale in a few hours" to be sure and call us in a few months when it went back on sale.

    d. Sent a letter to Oprah suggesting that she not deal with serious psychiatric issues in a superficial and therefore possible damaging manner to her guests. I then proposed a group therapy format with

HOW TO SURVIVE MENOPAUSE
WITHOUT GOING CRAZY

a real psychiatrist or psychotherapist.

Needless to say, I was on a rampage that week. By the way, the food company sent me another box of the grahams that tasted as awful as that first box of cookies from hell. The department store miraculously received my order the day after I called. The carpet lady, assured me she would call back when the carpet we liked went back on sale. I never did hear from Oprah ... for some reason.

Almost every writer on the subject of menopause acknowledges the presence of irritability as a fairly common factor during menopause. Dr. Burnett, as I mentioned in Chapter 1, places irritability at the very top of the list of signs of menopause reported 92% of the time. Those few authors who chose to deal with the subject in a little more depth recognize that estrogen deprivation is once again the culprit.

Anxiety and irritability are related. In fact, one of the symptoms of anxiety disorder is "exaggerated startle reflex." I have never been as jumpy as I was for a short period before I started hormone replacement. I would literally leap a few inches from my chair at loud noises or unexpected appearances or voices.

In The Silent Passage, Gail Sheehy describes a 42-year-old menopausal woman as a "virtual powder keg". She goes on to discuss how brain sensors that control emotions may overreact when there is an "erratic production of either estrogen or progesterone."

Besides estrogen deprivation, Sheehy also talks about another major cause of irritability during menopause, Provera. Ms. Sheehy discusses at length her own battle with this drug. Provera is the progestin that is often given along with estrogen that causes the uterine lining to slough off, preventing a dangerous, precancerous buildup. I would never take estrogen without progestin despite having to tolerate some very PMS-like side effects for 10 days during the month. Irritability is to me, by far, one of the problematic side effects.

A third major cause of irritability is sleeplessness which was covered in the last chapter. We can expect that if we have been up all night, or if our

IMPATIENCE: ONLY ONE SIGN OF IRRITABILITY

sleep has been interrupted, we are going to be very irritable the next day. We must do all we can to assure ourselves of a good night's sleep.

The three major causes of irritability that are easily identified are lack of estrogen, Provera, and lack of sleep. But, what causes the assertiveness that we discussed earlier that many women experience for the first time during menopause?

We've talked about periods of irritability, those times when due to the causes just mentioned we do become very impatient. Not nearly the raving maniacs that we may expect to turn into at the stroke of menopause. But pretty explosive at times. Nothing that estrogen supplements, a good nights sleep, some relaxation or other time-out exercises won't remedy after a while. But, what about this other thing? This, coming into our own so to speak. Do we experience some sort of permanent personality change?

Few authors are even willing to acknowledge this increased degree of assertiveness and yes, even aggressiveness in some menopausal women. Oh, they talk about how easily frustrated we become, how demanding we suddenly appear, even how hysterical and rageful we seem at times. Most talk about life changes that are occurring around the time of menopause. But, what about personal changes?

* * * *

One of my most important decisions made during menopause was I was no longer going to be superwoman. I realized that there were things I could do and others I could not. Even better, I realized there were things I wanted to do and things I definitely did not want to do. For years, we decorated our Christmas tree in the traditional red and green using ornaments that our children had made over the years. Every year, I swore I would do something different. Every year my family made me feel so guilty for even thinking about destroying our family tradition, I always changed my mind and pulled out the old decorations. Every one was happy but me. Well, during the height of my menopausal emergence as an ornery and unpredictable lady, I went out and bought all new decorations. Angels. I bought lots and

HOW TO SURVIVE MENOPAUSE
WITHOUT GOING CRAZY

lots of angels. I bought them because they made me happy. My adult children were mortified by the idea of a purple and gold color scheme, but begrudgingly admitted that the tree was indeed beautiful.

Another major change during that same Christmas. I didn't cook unless I really felt like it. Every year I'd run myself ragged trying to plan and prepare three meals a day during the holidays when our children visited. This time, we ate out a lot. My husband or daughter cooked more meals than I did. That also made me extremely happy. I was not nearly as depressed during this particular holiday period as I usually am.

During menopause, I really did feel the need to look out for myself. I found I could do this without feeling selfish. I really don't know how many women this new-found assertiveness happens to. As I said, very few authors recognize it and even if they do, fail to acknowledge it even exists. I wasn't aware of my own change in this area when I sent out the questionnaire. One writer, Germaine Greer, in <u>The Change: Women, Aging and the Menopause</u>, discusses the issue at length. In fact, in one of the most moving passages in her book, she gives her own interpretation of this change at menopause:

"Let the Masters in Menopause congregate in luxury hotels all over the world to deliver and to hearken to papers on the latest astonishing discoveries about the decline of grip strength in menopause or the number of stromal cells in the fifty-year-old ovary, the woman herself is too busy to listen. She is climbing her own mountain, in search of her own horizon, after years of being absorbed in the struggles of others. The way is hard, and she stumbles many times, but for once no one is scrambling after her, begging her to turn back. The air grows thin, and she may often feel dizzy. Sometimes the weariness spreads from her aching bones to her heart and brain, but she knows that, when she has scrambled up this sheer obstacle, she will see how to handle the rest of her long life. Some will climb swiftly, others will tack back and forth on the lower slopes, but few will give up. The truth is that fewer women

IMPATIENCE: ONLY ONE SIGN OF IRRITABILITY

come to grief at this obstacle than at any other in the tempestuous lives, though it is one of the stiffest challenges they ever face. Their behavior may baffle those who have unthinkingly exploited them all their lives before, but it is important not to explain, not to apologize. The climacteric marks the end of apologizing."

Although I believe more women do feel grief at this time, perhaps more than Ms. Greer would care to acknowledge, I also believe she's right on target in her assessment of the menopausal or climacteric woman coming into her own at this time. Indeed, although she no longer is willing to accept the smallest piece of the cake as young Sharon so astutely articulated, she also is less likely to apologize for not doing so.

HOW TO SURVIVE MENOPAUSE WITHOUT GOING CRAZY

FORGETTFULNESS

CHAPTER 7

FORGETFULNESS

I was very much aware that my youngest sister, Judy, a newlywed in her early thirties, was trying to get pregnant. Therefore, I was so delighted when Judy, a great cat-lover, sent me a postcard depicting a beautiful Persian with three fluffy baby kittens, bearing the handwritten message, "I thought I'd break it to you gently. Love, Judy."

I was so excited, I called Judy immediately to offer my congratulations and was very surprised and somewhat confused to learn that she was not pregnant. Instead, Judy explained that by sending the card, she was trying to find a kind way to tell me I was losing my memory without hurting my feelings too much.

A few months earlier, in response to her request for a donation to her favorite charity, I had sent Judy a check with a note explaining that the reason for such a "small" contribution was because I preferred to continue to support my own favorite charities instead. On the phone the day I called to congratulate her, Judy said she could certainly appreciate any donation no matter how small. But, since she searched long and hard for a check in my envelope with no success, she thought my contribution of zilch was a little bit too "small."

Anyway, she was reluctant to say anything about my lapse in memory until one of my other sisters told her that "all menopausal women are forgetful" and I would appreciate knowing about my

53

HOW TO SURVIVE MENOPAUSE
WITHOUT GOING CRAZY

shortcomings in the area. Actually, I didn't need the reminder.

Are all menopausal women forgetful? When I asked women to respond on my questionnaire whether or not they were forgetful during menopause, several cleverly responded, "I forget." However, almost all the respondents acknowledged they did experience forgetfulness during menopause. This was not surprising, since we all find ourselves from time to time walking into a room and forgetting what it was we set out to do only moments earlier. During menopause, this may happen so often, we can become alarmed. Are we getting Alzheimer's? By the way, in his book, *Menopause: All Your Questions Answered*, Raymond G. Burnett, M.D. cites at least one study that links estrogen deficiency to Alzheimer's. As in most matters relating to menopause, more research is indicated. But all of the most recent research on estrogen and Alzheimer's shows that the hormone not only helps in preventing the disease, but it can even restore lost mental abilities.

We do know for sure that the memory loss associated with menopause is in most cases, a temporary condition affecting a woman's short term memory. Not only may we forget why we've entered a particular room, but we often misplace things such as our keys or our glasses. Sometimes we cannot remember if we've turned off the stove or lowered the garage door. We may need to make several trips to the grocery store, since we can no longer depend on our mental list of items we need. We may double book our social calendars, forgetting that we've already committed to one engagement before accepting another. While I was writing this, I remembered something else we often forget, but it isn't in my notes and now I can't remember what it is. This is the absolute truth. Anyway, we simply do not have the sharp, short-term memory we had prior to entering menopause. Why?

According to Gail Sheehy in *The Silent Passage*, memory loss and estrogen deprivation are related and estrogen "does help increase the blood flow to the brain." Wulf H. Utian, M.D. and Ruth S. Jacobowitz in *Managing Your Menopause* also affirm that "decreasing estrogen levels

FORGETFULNESS

were linked to changes in short-term memory." So, although a 5/25/93 CNN report of a study done at the University of San Diego said estrogen does not help improve memory (women in this study with or without estrogen showed the same degree of age-related memory loss), the general belief is estrogen levels are directly related to short-term memory function. In fact, in his book, *Menopause: All Your Questions Answered*, Raymond G. Burnett, M.D. found that forgetfulness occurred with a frequency of 64%, sixth in a list of the 14 most common complaints by menopausal women.

As I write this chapter, I have been taking estrogen for about two years. My short-term memory has indeed improved, despite the fact that I just played a round of golf without remembering to put on my golf shoes. I knew something was different, but didn't realize what until I started to change back to my tennis shoes after we had finished. I had never changed in the first place. I had a good laugh. But, besides laughing at yourself and trying not to worry because you now know that most menopausal women become increasingly forgetful, what else can you do?

Until that estrogen replacement kicks in or if for medical or other reasons you decide not to take estrogen, there are ways to minimize memory problems. Some good advice comes from Kenneth L. Higbee, Ph.D. in *Your Memory: How It Works and How to Improve It*. He says, "If you want to remember something, you must pay attention to it, concentrate on it, and make sure you get it in the first place." His recommendation to pay attention in the first place if we want to remember something is especially meaningful to menopausal women who have trouble concentrating. (See Chapter 9) So, we do need to make an effort to focus our attention. As you pull out of the garage, make yourself visualize that garage door going down. When you take your glasses off or place your keys in a certain spot, take the time to see that place and fix it in your mind. Tell yourself, "I am putting my keys on the kitchen table." Better yet, place your keys, glasses, etc. in the same place every time. Take your hormones at the same time every day. I always put a patch out on the bathroom vanity

HOW TO SURVIVE MENOPAUSE
WITHOUT GOING CRAZY

the night before. Because I changed patches the first thing in the morning, if it was still sitting there the next day, I'd know I'd forgotten to put it on.

A key word for menopausal women is *organize*. We really do need to organize our lives at this time. Make lists for everything, not just for trips to the grocer. Use appointment books and refer to them daily to make sure you don't forget important birthdays and other occasions. Better yet, keep a calendar large enough for you to write reminders to yourself on or close to your phone.

There are lots of things we can do to help improve our memory. Use the so-called mnemonic "tricks" such as the ones we were taught in grade school to help us learn and remember certain things like how to spell Mississippi. One of my favorite mnemonic devices I still use to this day helps me recall how many days are in each month:

"Thirty days has September, April, June, and November..." You can find any of these association type aides in any book on memory. Keeping your mind active helps also. Read a lot. Do crossword puzzles, watch Jeopardy.

Once again, it is so important for us to remember that short-term memory problems associated with menopause is only a transient thing. Do not worry that you are losing your memory permanently, or that you are developing Alzheimer's. Like almost every other bane of menopause, this, too, will pass. Perhaps not completely, because as we get older, our memory lapses will increase. But, as long as forgetfulness doesn't interfere with our everyday functioning in life, then most experts agree we should not worry about it.

CHAPTER 8

FATIGUE

Dion, a 46-year-old insulin-dependent diabetic, has been on Premarin since her hysterectomy for unusually heavy periods a couple of years ago. She feels tired almost daily. She is pretty sure the fatigue is related to estrogen levels rather than blood sugar levels. Dion sums it up for all of us when she says, "I feel drained, physically and emotionally. When do these symptoms disappear? How long will I have to take the hormones?"

Dion's summation of her condition reflects the feeling of many of us. We are tired. Although this chapter focuses on the lethargy and fatigue some of us experience during menopause, perhaps, on an even broader level what we are really saying is we are tired of being menopausal.

What is to be made of the so-called lethargy that many menopausal women experience? The overwhelming fatigue that is both a physical and mental thing? The lack of motivation? The difficulty getting up and dragging ourselves off to work or just starting our day? The feeling tired all day? What happened to that "zest for life" that Margaret Mead said to expect after the change?

As we discussed in Chapter 4, fatigue may be one sign of clinical or serious depression. But very few women suffer major depression during menopause and almost all experience fatigue during this time. In fact, Raymond Burnett, M.D. in *Menopause: All Your Questions Answered*, lists lethargy/fatigue as the second most reported sign of menopause at

HOW TO SURVIVE MENOPAUSE
WITHOUT GOING CRAZY

88%. And in *The Silent Passage: Menopause*, Gail Sheehy mentions having "little crashes of fatigue" herself. And almost everyone who responded to my own menopause survey listed fatigue as one of the symptoms experienced at least once a month.

Fatigue during menopause could be related to several causes. The most obvious is sleeplessness. For so many of us, it is not unusual to feel rotten if we've only had a few hours sleep the night before. Fatigue in perimenopause, especially, could be due to excessive bleeding. It is always wise to have your doctor check to make sure you are not anemic. Although my gynecologist believes anemia due to heavy periods has to be rare due to the many supplements available to women today. And as we've mentioned, severe depression may be the culprit for a few of us. There are certainly other reasons, unrelated to menopause, for fatigue. Much is being made of the fact, for example, that light deprivation causes fatigue. It won't hurt to make sure you get enough light through natural or artificial means if necessary. However, once again if you're perimenopausal and you're feeling tired, it's not unusual.

It is possible the lethargy we feel might also be related to the fact that suffering through a long, difficult menopause is literally getting us down. Feeling low, anxious, sleepy, and irritable can be tiring. We find ourselves extending a tremendous amount of energy just trying to feel good. I can remember trying to explain this lack of vitality to my husband when even the simplest task seemed like a major chore. You would have thought he had asked to go mountain climbing once by my incredulously violent reaction to a simple request that I make us a cup of tea. "I'm exhausted," I must have said hundreds of times for a couple of years.

So do we just have to wait til we're post menopausal to regain the energy that we had prior to menopause? To feel that "post-menopausal zest" the famous anthropologist talked about? Of course, it's interesting to note that Margaret Mead was taking estrogen injections at the time of her own menopause. In fact, according to Gail Sheehy, Mead took estrogen from age 48 until she reached her sixties.

FATIGUE

It makes sense that estrogen replacement will help to restore lost energy. First of all, HRT, can help stabilize irregular, heavy bleeding in the perimenopausal woman. Next, estrogen replacement almost always relieves hot flashes which we know is a major reason our sleep is disturbed at night. Therefore, when considering whether or not to take hormones, relief from fatigue is another major consideration.

In *Managing Your Menopause*, Wulf H. Utian, M.D. and Ruth S. Jacobowitz discuss the role of estrogen in the revitalization of some menopausal women. The women in Dr. Utian's practice are described as feeling "more alert and better able to function." The authors also discuss the importance of exercise in producing a feeling of well-being in the menopausal woman.

I have found exercise to be a major motivator during those times when I feel my energy dwindling. I know it sounds nuts to say when you're feeling too tired to walk to the next room, the best thing to do is walk a mile or so. But, it does help. I have developed my own exercise program based on what's fun for me. I exercise during the weekdays with either Denise or Gil on ESPN. I walk a mile in the morning and a mile in the afternoon. I lift weights for a few minutes at least three times a week. Exercise releases endorphins, a brain chemical that is known to enhance feelings of well-being. I can't emphasize enough how important exercise is. But, you need to develop your own program. I can't stand the stationary bike, but most of my friends love it. I have never been on a treadmill, yet my Mom, who is in her seventies, uses her daily. So, walk, bike, run, buy a Jane Fonda tape, but keep on moving if you want to keep your energy level up. Be sure and discuss any exercise program with your doctor before you start. But start.

To Dion and all of us who are "physically and emotionally drained," I wish we could see ahead to that time when we no longer yearn for the vigor of our pre-menopausal days. Perhaps there is an increased energy, that certain "zest" that Margaret Mead talked about somewhere down the road. According to Ms. Sheehy, at least, there does exist a vitality that some

HOW TO SURVIVE MENOPAUSE
WITHOUT GOING CRAZY

post-menopausal women begin to experience in their mid-fifties. I, for one, can't wait.

INABILITY TO CONCENTRATE

CHAPTER 9

INABILITY TO CONCENTRATE

Louise has always been dedicated to staying youthful looking and attractive. Like most of us, she's somewhat surprised that she's old enough to be menopausal. She opted for taking only small doses of replacement hormones because of a tendency to develop breast cysts. Generally, she seems to be taking menopause in stride despite experiencing several of the more unpleasant menopausal symptoms such as her fearful awakening at night mentioned in Chapter 6.

Two of the symptoms she didn't even know were associated with menopause are very amusing to her. "I itch," she laughs. "Itch?" I asked. "You mean the creepy-crawly feeling a lot of women get during menopause?" (See Chapter 10) "Not really," she responded. "I just itch, especially under my armpits." After a few jokes about changing deodorants, Louise discussed one of the other humorous, but somewhat more worrisome symptoms of menopause that had appeared at the onset of her perimenopause.

Louise has difficulty "hearing" what others are saying. "I'm not talking about a hearing problem," she explains, "or the fact that it's hard for me to hear if there's a lot of noise. But, someone will be talking to me and I simply don't know what they have just said." "In fact," she continues, "my sister has the same problem. And, it's not that I try to shut people out. I just lose track of what they're saying."

HOW TO SURVIVE MENOPAUSE
WITHOUT GOING CRAZY

Louise's complaint is a common one among menopausal women. Feeling distracted, foggy thinking, inability to concentrate or becoming confused are just some of the ways women describe this curious phenomenon.

Quite a few experts have discussed memory loss or forgetfulness during menopause as I discovered when researching Chapter 7. However, I found little or no information on the loss of concentration or the diminished ability to concentrate that so many women also experience during this time. Most authors tend to discuss this problem with concentration along with forgetfulness, as though the two are the same. And, although closely related (you could certainly forget what you walked into a certain room to get if you were distracted), I believe we're dealing with two distinct problems.

* * * *

One day I was getting dressed to go out and couldn't find a favorite pair of gold earrings. I looked in the usual places and then everywhere I could possibly imagine with no luck. I was heartbroken because those earrings were a gift from my son and were very special to me. But after searching for a couple of days with no luck, I gave up and accepted the fact that I had lost them. Then, one day I was in the bathroom putting on makeup when I glanced down and saw one of the earrings nestled in the carpet. I had looked repeatedly in that same area during my search and knew that the earring had not been there before. In fact, I had even vacuumed the area. I rushed to check the vacuum cleaner bag to see if the other earring was in it but I couldn't find it. Then, I remembered that I had emptied the little trash can into a garbage bag earlier. Perhaps it had fallen to the floor in the process. I rushed to check the garbage bag, but still could not find the other earring. Then, in a rare flash of brilliance, I checked the bottom of the trash can and sure enough, stuck in the corner was my other gold earring. You can't imagine how relieved I was to find that earring until I realized that I had obviously thrown my precious earrings into the trash. Now that's scary. Memory loss? Not hardly.

INABILITY TO CONCENTRATE

Distracted? To say the least. Almost as bad as the time I tried to stuff the flagpole into my golf bag instead of my putter. My golf partner was looking at me as if I'd really gone batty, but I still didn't realize what I was doing till she burst out laughing. It was funny.

When conducting the survey of menopausal women, I found that several admitted to experiencing both forgetfulness and inability to concentrate while some reported only forgetfulness. But interestingly enough, *almost all* indicated they had trouble concentrating during menopause. So, why has so little attention been given to the matter? Perhaps because the subject of absent-mindedness has always been amusing. This is one symptom of menopause that doesn't send us running off to see our doctors, even our psychiatrists. In fact, once we know that it is just one other strange, but innocuous and temporary aberration to be tolerated as we struggle through menopause, many of us can and do laugh at ourselves and the tragic comedies we find ourselves starring in.

About five years ago I gave up smoking after over 20 years of indulging in this pleasurable, but self-destructive habit. One of the major side-effects of nicotine withdrawal that was particularly bothersome to me was a sudden inability to concentrate. I simply could not stay focused on anything longer than a few minutes at a time. I couldn't read. I couldn't watch TV. What I experienced at that time is very similar to what women experience during menopause. I don't believe any research has been done to determine the cause. We do know that nicotine affects adrenaline and dopamine in the brain. And, according to Tom Fergerson, M.D. in *The No-Nag, No-Guilt, Do-It-Your-Own-Way Guide to Quitting Smoking*, nicotine does seem "to help smokers feel less overwhelmed by disruptive or distracting stimulation in their environment and makes it easier for them to concentrate on the task at hand." Estrogen, like nicotine, affects these same brain chemicals. So, maybe someday, someone will discover that estrogen withdrawal has something to do with our changing from clear-thinking individuals to somewhat flaky women for at least one brief moment

HOW TO SURVIVE MENOPAUSE
WITHOUT GOING CRAZY

in our lives.

Once again, not knowing the cause of our sudden confused and distracted state of mind does not mean that we simply must tolerate the situation til we emerge from menopause. There are steps we can take to come through the fog without any major misfortunes occurring. Except for maybe throwing away one of our favorite pieces of jewelry or stealing a flag-pole from the golf course. And, as I told Louise about her inability to concentrate on what others are saying to her, "Sometimes, it is helpful to tune out certain people who make demands on your time and energy. Especially, when it is taking all you have just to get through menopause." In other words, maybe the inability to concentrate is really a coping mechanism in disguise.

Despite my somewhat cavalier attitude toward this particular symptom of menopause, it is still a problem that should not be dismissed lightly, and the question of what to do about it needs to be addressed. And first of all, like all of the problems associated with menopause discussed so far, the first step toward alleviation of the problem is recognition that it exists. So don't panic when your concentration goes. Remember, it is a temporary inconvenience that will disappear as you pass over to the other side of menopause.

Another helpful solution to the issue of diminishing ability to think clearly is to concentrate on concentration. In other words, practice concentrating on one thing at a time. Whether it's a favorite TV program or book, or puzzle, when you find your mind drifting, make yourself focus on what you're doing at the moment. When you feel yourself losing tract or interest, force yourself to refocus on what you're doing. The same applies when listening. Make yourself refocus as soon as you recognize that you're no longer hearing what another is saying to you.

It is important to recognize the connection between sleep deprivation and the inability to concentrate the next day. So, doing all you can to get a decent night's sleep as discussed in Chapter 5, will also go a long way in reducing concentration problems. And, as we saw in Chapter 6, getting a

INABILITY TO CONCENTRATE

good night's sleep will also make it easier to deal with that other prevalent but barely discussed symptom of menopause, irritability.

While you're waiting for your ability to concentrate to return, don't forget that humor goes a long way in making things better. Laugh at yourself a little. Like I did not too long ago while shopping at my favorite little grocery store. I was pushing a shopping cart when I stopped to search for my usual after-dinner mints. Unable to find them, I proceeded down the aisles to get the other things on my shopping list. It wasn't until two aisles and several quizzical smiles from other shoppers later, did I realize I was pushing a cart full of discontinued candy instead of my regular assortment of healthy foods. "My husband has a sweet tooth," I mumbled to one gentleman who asked if I liked candy. Talk about being distracted. But, it was so funny, I began to laugh as I walked away. Out loud. Eliciting even more stares.

HOW TO SURVIVE MENOPAUSE WITHOUT GOING CRAZY

CREEPY-CRAWLY FEELINGS & OTHER WEIRD HAPPENINGS

CHAPTER 10

CREEPY-CRAWLY FEELINGS & OTHER WEIRD HAPPENINGS

One night I was sitting on the sofa watching one of the sitcoms when my scalp started moving. I felt like little bugs were having a party under my scalp. "Wow," I thought, "I must not have rinsed the hair color out of my hair well enough." "But that's ridiculous," I argued with myself, "I've been using the same hair product for years and nothing like this has ever happened." The weird sensation lasted several minutes and scared me to death. I had heard of similar reactions from patients who were undergoing withdrawal from either alcohol or certain other drugs. I even knew the name for this strange phenomenon, formication. Please note, I said <u>formication</u>. Anyway, I had no idea why this horrible feeling thing was happening to me. It was months before it happened again, this time in a movie theater. A pulling across the skin on my left arm. I had told my husband about the first episode, using the hair color explanation so he would not think I was crazy. I decided to tell him about the second one also, simply because I needed verification that I was not going crazy. Despite not knowing what was really going on with me, he did reassure me that I still was lucid. I experienced the creepy-crawly feelings only one other time, but by then, I had a name for what was occurring and I had already started taking hormones. It never happened again.

HOW TO SURVIVE MENOPAUSE
WITHOUT GOING CRAZY

Once, I started looking, I found several authors who at least mentioned formication as a symptom of menopause. Lately it seems everyone who is well versed in the matter of menopause acknowledges that it does indeed exist.

Dr. Lila Nachtigill in her book, <u>Estrogen: The Facts Can Save Your Life</u>, has a somewhat lengthy discussion of the unusual occurance: "Undoubtedly the strangest, and often the most frightening, menopausal symptom of all is formication, a crawling feeling over the skin. Luckily, this is fairly rare. One patient recently thought she was having an emotional breakdown because of these odd sensations and like everyone else who gets this one was enormously relieved to find out it is a typical, though infrequent menopausal occurrance."

Dr. Nachtigall verifies what I learned by accident, that these sensations of insects crawling under one's skin are relieved by estrogen. And if estrogen replacement relieves the symptom, it is obviously caused by estrogen deprivation in the first place.

It is hard to describe this peculiar sensation or to even try to tell you just how scary it is to actually experience it. I looked formication up in Stedman's Medical Dictionary recently. It was defined as "a form of paresthesia or tactile hallucination in which one feels a sensation as of small insects creeping under the skin, usually seen in substance induced organic mental syndromes." Believe me, then, when I say, that this symptom of menopause more than any other can cause you to believe that you might be losing your sanity. And having formication described as a "tactile hallucination" doesn't help either. Since we all know having hallucinations doesn't exactly mean we're in the best mental health. Since most menopausal women don't even know that formication exists and that it is related to estrogen deprivation, experiencing it can be dreadful. Most medical dictionaries define formication, I am happy to report, as paresthesia, an altered sensation in the skin that causes numbness or tingling. One resource actually distinguishes it from paranoid delusions which made me feel a whole lot better.

CREEPY-CRAWLY FEELINGS & OTHER WEIRD HAPPENINGS

Thankfully, these creepy-crawly feelings are rare. Of the fifty or so women I questioned about this particular symptom, only three said they had experienced it. I was one of the unlucky ones who did. Of course, as you may be beginning to realize by now, I had it all! If you also are unfortunate enough to have to endure these sensations, remember that it's just one other sign of menopause. These awful sensations will last only a few minutes. Try to relax. You'll have the impulse to scratch. Don't, because you can really irritate the skin. I know I found myself rubbing the area in a gentle massage and this seemed to help a little. At least psychologically. But, most importantly, try not to be afraid. This, too, will pass. In *Estrogen: Is It Right For You?*, Paula Dranov says that the skin tingling could continue for years, but like everyone else, she also reports that taking estrogen helps.

Besides formication, some women complain of other lessor known symptoms during menopause. My own well-informed gynecologist told me his patients have complained of most of these unusual signs of menopause. But, a couple of them even he had never heard of. I believe this is because they are so strange we simply do not associate them with menopause so we don't mention them to our doctors. We don't want them to think we're nuts. Among these other weird happenings are: headaches, a tingling, pins and needles feeling or numbness in the arms, weak spells, dizziness, shortness of breath, nausea, being bothered by loud noise or sharp smells.

The first two, headaches and parethesia, are really not that surprising when you consider that like formication and hot flashes, they involve the vascular system. The relationship between menopause and vasomotor problems although well established, has, like almost everything else to do with the change, very little scientific research to explain it.

A very dear friend of mine thought she was having a stroke or heart attack when periodically, she felt a numbness in her arm. I told her about my discovering the connection between parethesia and menopause as I did the research for this book. I also encouraged her to see her physician, since many of the signs of menopause may indeed be caused by something else.

HOW TO SURVIVE MENOPAUSE
WITHOUT GOING CRAZY

I will talk further about this matter of how to determine if your problems are related to menopause or to some other cause later on in the chapter. Anyway, my friend was extremely relieved to learn that this numbness might be related to menopause instead of to serious heart problems as she had first believed. After a while on estrogen, the worrisome symptom just went away. It's also interesting to note that when questioned about this particular sign, several women responded that they did indeed feel numbness in their arms at least once a month.

Weakness and dizziness have been frequently reported by menopausal women. These symptoms could also be related to the vascular system. We know that fainting is usually due to a decrease in blood flow to the brain. Even having cold hands and feet which is sometimes mentioned as a menopausal symptom, might result from vascular problems.

Although we do not fully understand the role estrogen plays in relation to these symptoms associated with the vascular system, we do know that estrogen directly affects the lining of blood vessels and that estrogen replacement does work to relieve all of them. By the way, as mentioned in the chapter on fatigue, weakness could possibly be related to anemia due to heavier than normal bleeding during perimenopause, but this is not likely.

* * * *

One summer during the height of my menopausal woes, my sister and her husband attended a convention in San Antonio where we lived. They invited my husband and me to attend two dinner functions with them. The first was an outdoor Mexican/Western buffet held at La Valita on the Riverwalk, one of my favorite spots in the city. I was looking forward to the event, but as soon as I arrived, the strong smells that I had always associated with delicious Mexican food and great Texan barbecue made me so nauseated I thought I was going to embarrass myself in front of several hundred people. I immediately thought the nausea was caused by the anxiety that I had begun to have on several occasions when we went out to dinner.

However, we went out to dinner again the next night. This time

CREEPY-CRAWLY FEELINGS & OTHER WEIRD HAPPENINGS

to a gourmet meal at a wonderful museum in San Antonio. The meal was great. No nausea. No anxiety. What was the difference, I wondered.

The difference I learned later is I was not having hot flashes on the second night in question. The hot summer night, the stress I had now begun to associate with going out, had set off a series of hot flashes. It wasn't til much later I learned that there was indeed a connection between nausea and hot flashes.

I read about an interesting study in Paula Dravnov's *Estrogen: Is It Right For You?* Ms. Dravnov discusses the work of Fredi Kronenberg, a researcher at Columbia studying hot flashes. When asking her menopausal subjects to describe their hot flashes, Kronenberg found that 57.8% experienced nausea. In fact, the symptom of nausea during hot flashes was reported more often than any other problem, including embarrassment and anxiety.

I have been unable to learn what causes the nausea during the hot flash. I do know there is a relationship between nausea and anxiety and as discussed earlier in the chapter on hot flashes, anxiety is usually present during the flash. I had complained for a couple of years that strong smells literally made me sick. I attributed this problem to the fact that I smoked for 25 years and when I stopped and could suddenly smell again, the smells were so overwhelming, they often made me nauseated. My poor daughter has had to make several adjustments to her erratic menopausal Mom. She loves perfumes, but has learned to stay away from me or go lightly on the sweet stuff because of my sensitivity to it.

I firmly believe there is a strong connection between hot flashes, strong smells, and nausea. Therefore the best way to handle the nausea is to handle the hot flash. (See Chapter 2) Other than that, carry lots of Pepto-Bismal tablets. Or make sure you're taking your calcium. Besides it being practically mandatory that you get enough calcium during menopause to prevent osteoporosis, calcium has also been found to be helpful in calming that queasy stomach.

HOW TO SURVIVE MENOPAUSE
WITHOUT GOING CRAZY

Several sources have made the observation that menopausal women are often bothered by loud noise. This was one of the symptoms my gynecologist had not heard of. But noise can, in fact, set off a hot flash. We talked about being hypersensitive to noise and the so-called "startle reflex" in Chapter 6. Having an exaggerated startle reflex is one sign of anxiety disorder. So, once again, it's not surprising to find a connection between hot flashes, anxiety, and loud noises. And once again, the main solution seems to be to try to eliminate the hot flashes.

There have been mention of numerous other rare symptoms during menopause. Shortness of breath is one. Feelings of suffocation, another. Both obviously related to anxiety and the hot flash. One source even listed visual defects such as difficulty reading road signs as being related to menopause.

So many symptoms! And, I sometimes feel as if I had every single one of them. How do we know all of these problems are really related to menopause? I used to think that maybe I was less emotionally stable than I thought. Surely, going through a natural transitional state could not be causing such emotional turmoil. Like Kate in Chapter 4 who questions whether or not her depression is really connected to her menopause, we may find that we're just not sure that it's not just "all in our heads" as we've been told forever.

A good indicator of what's actually happening, I believe, is to take an honest, objective look at yourself. If you are experiencing an early menopause because of surgery. Or if you are between the ages of 45 and 55 and have never had these problems before, there's a good chance they are related to menopause. If you are in the perimenopause phase and your periods are irregular, but have not stopped completely, these symptoms, once again, are probably related to menopause. If you're not sure you're in the perimenopausal stage, the following physical signs may indicate that you are: Irregular, heavy, light, or absent periods, vaginal tightness, painful intercourse, often accompanied by decreased sexual desire, urinary incontinence, and especially the almost always present hot flash.

CREEPY-CRAWLY FEELINGS & OTHER WEIRD HAPPENINGS

If some of the physical changes are taking place because of abnormally low or fluctuating hormone levels, then don't be surprised that some of the emotional problems are also appearing for the first time in your life for the same reason.

HOW TO SURVIVE MENOPAUSE WITHOUT GOING CRAZY

FEARFULNESS

CHAPTER 11

FEARFULNESS

I've always thought of myself as a brave person. And, as I approached menopause, I was not scared at all. In fact, I simply did not think about it. Maybe that's why I became so frightened by what began happening to both my body and my mind. While outwardly, I tried to appear courageous and strong, I was slowly beginning to feel like a sniveling coward.

I am a nurse. I should have been prepared for menopause, but I was not. Like most women, I had no idea what to expect. My aunt who is in her seventies told me how frustrating it was for her when she went through "the change." "No one told us what to expect in those days. We didn't know what to do about it because we just didn't talk about menopause when I went through it. I had a terrible time, but I just had to suffer in silence. It was pretty scary."

Not knowing what to expect or having horrible expectations based on old wives' tales passed down from one generation to another are the main causes of fear about menopause. The unknown always makes us uneasy as we all know. Even in the 90's, we are still not prepared for the changes that are about to occur as we enter the perimenopausal (the three to five years before menses actually ceases) stage of life.

HOW TO SURVIVE MENOPAUSE
WITHOUT GOING CRAZY

Once perimenopause has begun, fear surrounding menopause is usually associated with the following:

1. The sudden appearance of irregular and/or very heavy bleeding. Skipping periods for a couple of months, followed by ones that are unusually long. You may have been fairly regular before, but now you don't know what to expect. Having a well-meaning physician tell you the excessive bleeding could be caused by cancer rather than reassuring you that it's probably due to fluctuating hormone levels during perimenopause.

2. Experiencing other disturbing physical changes, especially, vaginal dryness/tightness, resulting in painful intercourse and diminished sexual drive. Having to deal with incontinence or frequent urination which almost always occurs during menopause.

3. Increasingly frequent thoughts of aging and death. Feeling old, fat, unattractive, fatigued. Concern about losing your youthful appearance and energy. I actually thought my upper lip was getting thinner. Maybe it was.

4. The appearance of some really unusual menopausal signs such as formication (the sensation of insects crawling under your skin) and numbness in your arms.

5. The fairly traumatic things that can happen during hot flashes: anxiety, nausea, embarrassment.

6. Worry about whether or not you should take hormones. Will they cause cancer? Make you fatter? Depressed?

7. The sudden moodiness, tearfulness that makes us wonder if we are indeed going crazy.

When and if some of these things begin happening to you, there are steps you can take to make the situation less frightening:

1. Check out unusual periods; absent, heavy or irregular bleeding. Tell your physician you suspect you're menopausal. He or she may suggest a FSH (follicle stimulating hormone) blood test, telling you that if this level is high, you're menopausal. If it is below a certain level, you are not. Remind your doctor that even if it is still low, you are experiencing other

FEARFULNESS

symptoms of menopause. Talk to your physician about the perimenopausal stage of the change and the fluctuating hormone levels that occur at this time. Keep in mind many physicians, even gynecologists are still not well-informed about menopause. So, if your doctor has never heard of perimenopause, get out of his office as fast as you can and find another one. Because my periods had not stopped and my FSH level was still low, the first gynecologist I saw told me I was not menopausal. According to this same doctor, the heavy, prolonged bleeding I was experiencing was not normal. That's when a very painful endometrial biopsy was performed to see if I had cancer. I was terrified.

If you have unusual bleeding, your physician may suggest an endometrial biopsy to rule out other causes for it besides menopause. You certainly want to consider undergoing this 15 to 20 minute office procedure. The doctor may tell you it's a little uncomfortable as mine did. That's an understatement. For most women, this "uncomfortable" sampling of the uterine lining hurts. A lot. But, it's worth the pain if the test comes back negative for endometrial cancer. Definitely opt for the office biopsy before submitting to hospital surgery. Far too many unnecessary hysterectomies are still being performed today. And, some women actually want them because the heavy bleeding is so frightening for them. Irregular bleeding can be controlled by hormones. Talk to your physician about the possibility. If he or she tells you that since your menses hasn't completely stopped, you shouldn't take hormones, get a second opinion or a third, if that's what it takes.

2. So many women entering menopause are afraid that their sex lives will soon be over. Although there is no proof that sexual drive is lower during and following menopause, it is a fact that painful intercourse due to vaginal dryness and tightness can certainly put a damper on your enthusiasm for sex. Lovemaking that hurts is not fun. And sex that is not pleasurable, isn't going to do wonders for your libido. The fear resulting from menopausal tightness can be devastating. Fear of the actual pain. Fear that you may bleed during intercourse. Fear that you will lose all interest in sex.

HOW TO SURVIVE MENOPAUSE
WITHOUT GOING CRAZY

Fear that your sexual partner won't understand. Or that he will lose his desire for you. There are several things you can do to remedy the situation. First, talk with your physician about hormone replacement therapy. You will notice an almost miraculous return to normal very shortly. If you can't take hormones or choose not to, you might want to try a vaginal cream or moisturizer. Estrogen replacement will also help restore bladder control. For those women who choose not to go the hormone replacement route, Kegel exercises to strengthen the vaginal muscles can be tried. Talk to your physician about all of these situations.

It is very important that while you are attempting to remedy the situation in regards to possible deteriorating sexual relations, you need to make your sexual partner aware of what's happening to your body. He may need reassurance that your reluctance at times to engage in sexual activity is a temporary thing brought on by the changes in your body and that you still find him sexually attractive. If you do, that is. He may become less amorous also, particularly if he's afraid of hurting you. Especially after he realizes your screams during intercourse are not exactly your usual cries of ecstasy. Anyway, make your mate a partner in every sense of the word. He should be included in all aspects of your menopausal passage, especially the difficult sexual period that you may go through. The only way our loved ones can help us deal with the fear surrounding menopause is if we share it with them

3. Fear associated with aging is often present at the time of menopause. I read a novel recently in which the heroine in her late forties was really distraught over the fact that men did not turn their heads when she walked by as they used to. It's kind of like looking in the mirror and discovering that your upper lip is disappearing while you're developing a ball under your chin. The fact that my face began changing, especially when my chin line started going away, was one of the most difficult things for me to accept. Not the weight gain. I had learned to control that when I gave up smoking and put on lots of extra pounds. A healthy, low fat diet and exercise are the key to keeping your body in shape. But you can't exercise your face.

FEARFULNESS

Well, actually, there are supposed to be facial exercises that can help the sagging. The concept is new, however, and still unproven. But, there's cosmetic surgery for the more adventurous among us and hair and facial makeovers for those of us less enamored of pain. What else? Drink lots of water, stop smoking and wrinkling at the same time. Treat yourself to a massage, a facial, a manicure at your favorite spa or beauty salon. Most importantly, make friends with the new you. The older model may not be as beautiful as the younger one, but it can certainly be attractive. I used to hate that word, but I have learned that terms such as *attractiveness, sexy, youthful* are all relative. You are what you believe yourself to be. So do what you can to enhance that skinny upper lip, then forget it. Chances are it still turns your mate on. The fear of aging need not be paralyzing. Use that fear to mobilize yourself to action in pursuit of the new and better you.

    4. Be prepared for the possibility of some really unusual vascular things happening during perimenopause. You may have headaches, numbness or tingling in your arms (parathesia), or the rare but terrifying formication. It is really scary to experience the sensation of insects crawling under your skin. I thought I was hallucinating the first time it happened to me. You can imagine how relieved I was to learn that hormone deprivation caused the strange phenomenon and hormone replacement could get rid of it. If any of these signs of perimenopause appears, don't be afraid. As I said, many physicians are not yet well-informed about menopause. So, they fail to connect these symptoms to the change. But, our fears about the unusual signs of menopause can be lessened by a visit to a physician. If only to rule out serious disease such as heart attack or stroke for the woman who feels occasional numbness in her arms and imagines the worst. Chances are if you are menopausal, the decrease in estrogen is affecting your blood vessels, causing the above problems. So, don't be afraid.

    5. Just knowing that most of us are going to have hot flashes and that we are not alone when we feel the anxiety, nausea, discomfort, and embarrassment that goes along with them helps to alleviate the fear associated with them. It is also encouraging to know that hormone

HOW TO SURVIVE MENOPAUSE
WITHOUT GOING CRAZY

replacement is available to quickly relieve us of this other bane of menopause. For those of us who will not or cannot take hormones, try to stay as cool as possible to lessen the severity and frequency of the flash. Avoid hot foods, places, baths, weather. Most importantly, avoid stressful situations. Be encouraged by the knowledge that the hot flashes will not last forever.

6. The question of whether or not to take hormones can be very anxiety provoking. Most women don't like taking medication and are hesitant to ingest anything new and possibly alien to our bodies. Besides, we've heard that hormones can cause both breast and endometrial cancers. It's confusing: Warned to stop smoking because lighting up may cause cancer. Then told that although hormones may also cause cancer, it's OK to use them.

I believe we're afraid to take hormones, but at the same time, we're afraid not to take them. No one but you can make the decision about whether or not you should take hormone supplements. What you need to do is make an informed decision. Someone said our level of functioning after menopause will be different than it was prior to the change if we do not take hormones. We will not have the enhanced feelings of well-being that often accompanies hormone replacement. For many women, the somewhat lower level of functioning is the price they pay for not having to worry about the negative consequences of taking hormones. Most women do not even recognize or acknowledge that they are operating at a less than optimal status after menopause. For them, the only reason to take hormones is to prevent heart disease and/or osteoporosis, diseases related to estrogen deprivation after menopause. Research is still inconclusive about whether or not estrogen causes cancer. We know that so many symptoms of menopause will disappear almost as soon as we start hormone replacement. It angers me that it is the late 90's and I have to make a decision about taking hormones based on inadequate data. It also angers me that I have to be afraid to take a drug I know will help me. Hopefully, some of the fear associated with hormones will be eliminated after weighing

FEARFULNESS

the pros and cons of taking them. I just wish there were no cons.

7. Finally, the fear that arises from the mood changes that occur during perimenopause needs to be mentioned. When the tears begin flowing for no apparent reason, that's scary. It's also frightening when we're feeling happy and hopeful one moment and depressed and pessimistic soon after. We can wonder if we're going crazy when we are serene and calm one hour and irritable and violent the next. Our emotions are indeed on a virtual roller-coaster. Do not be afraid. Expect that some women will experience these things when their hormone levels start dropping. We undergo some pretty wild fluctuations in hormone levels during perimenopause that definitely affect our emotions. Despite the fact many in the medical profession deny a connection between depression and menopause, if you experience more than temporary blues, you should seek a professional opinion. Especially if your depression is interfering with your ability to function. Just remember, you are not going crazy. You are not alone. You will feel better.

So many reasons to be fearful during menopause. I was afraid of never feeling really good again. Both physically and emotionally. I still think a good deal about the premenopausal me. The woman who had very few fears. We are being told by the so-called authorities on the subject that menopause is not a disease, that we may have a few hot flashes, become a little irritable, but not to worry. It's just a phase. Well, menopause may be just a normal aspect of a woman' life, but we still have to know what to expect. Some very frightening things may happen to us and we need to be prepared.

I understand fear as I have never understood it before. I have always believed the mind controls the body. That you could pray or talk yourself out of illness, even serious ones. During the height of my perimenopausal woes, I spent a vast amount of time doing mental exercises to relax. Listening to Dr. Bernie Seigel's tapes became a daily routine for me. Now I am convinced mind and body affect each other. I can tell you, as I have several times and you can tell yourself, "Do not be afraid." But, when the

HOW TO SURVIVE MENOPAUSE
WITHOUT GOING CRAZY

adrenalin is coursing through your body during a hot flash-induced panic attack, your mind is not going to believe that all is well, no matter what you tell yourself. On the other hand, you can do things to relax the mind, thus minimizing the severity of the attack, and relieving the fearfulness associated with it and with menopause in general.

One of the most helpful exercises I've found to ward off an anxiety attack is very simple. It is a basic muscle relaxation tool that's been around forever. Start by making a fist, tensing for a few seconds, then relaxing the hand for the same amount of time. The idea is to tense, then relax major muscles in your body. After the hands, do the same routine with your arms, forehead, jaw, neck, shoulders, chest, abdomen, legs, feet and toes. The great thing about this relaxation technique is any part of it can be done anywhere, anytime. Even while you're driving. I've always found a dark theater especially conducive to its practice.

In the next chapter, I'll mention another couple of mental exercises from my favorite panic attack book that I've found helpful during those times when fear overtook me and made me feel so powerless. Being afraid had become a way of life for me, but I have been able to overcome most of my irrational fears. I said most of them. I'm still afraid of flying. I fly, but I'll never be a happy flyer. I suppose I never was. Even before menopause.

ACHIEVING GOOD MENTAL HEALTH DURING MENOPAUSE

CHAPTER 12

ACHIEVING GOOD MENTAL HEALTH DURING MENOPAUSE

I went to my nephew's wedding recently. Actually, I flew to my nephew's wedding. I was anxious the night before, but I flew drug free. OK. So it was only an hour's flight from Dallas to Memphis. The thing is I flew, I attended the wedding and reception, gambled at Tunica, went to Graceland, and I didn't have one moment of panic. I had fun. "Is that when you know you're post-menopausal?" I asked myself. "When you start having fun again?"

I made it through menopause without going crazy. You can't imagine how happy I am to repeat those words. I made it through menopause. It didn't just happen suddenly. I mean, it wasn't like one morning I woke up and said, "I'm post-menopausal." It ended the same way it started. For me it was a slow and very painful journey. In *Estrogen: The Facts Can Change Your Life*, Dr. Lila Nachtigall discusses some of the emotional things that happen to us during menopause. She describes the emotional component as an "early symptom" that "almost always fades away in less than a year." Wouldn't that be wonderful? The fact is the symptoms peak during perimenopause and we know that this stage of the change can last as long as 10 years.

In my case, perimenopause was a five or six year process that seemed at times as if it would never end. But, it did. Somewhere along the way I would go whole months without a hot flash. I can't remember when I

HOW TO SURVIVE MENOPAUSE
WITHOUT GOING CRAZY

stopped throwing the covers off at night. Or when I began to be able to tolerate the heat generated by my husband's body as he reached out for me in his sleep. One day I realized I was actually cold when it was cold outside.

Panic attacks were a terrifying residual effect of menopause for me. I learned how to handle them by reading and applying everything I could get my hands on about the disorder and by praying a lot. I haven't had one in ages. I am no longer moody. I remember things. I'm less tired. I don't have all that wonderful energy, the so-called zest for life that Margaret Mead talked about, but I don't suppose I had it even before menopause. However, I'm no longer exhausted all the time and that's a major accomplishment.

I still have trouble sleeping. I fall asleep right away, but I often find myself awake in the early morning hours even though the hot flashes that once woke me in the middle of the night are long gone. I've developed a routine that works for me. I get up, read or write. Often I watch T.V. The weather channel soothes me and puts me back to sleep. No plot there for me to become involved with. Sometimes I go back to bed. Sometimes I don't. It doesn't matter. Since I usually feel fine the next day, I know I'm getting enough sleep.

I'm no longer mean or impatient with others. In fact, I have become a kinder, more sensitive person all around. I suppose the biggest post-menopausal change has to do with the fearfulness that had incapacitated me for so long. I am no longer afraid.

I have said often enough how much I yearned to be my pre-menopausal self. Am I? I don't think so. If going through menopause is indeed progressing through a natural phase of life as most women believe, then we know we can expect some growth to take place. Menopause was not easy for me. But, I learned compassion for other women who are not having an easy time of it. As a nurse, I didn't think I needed to learn empathy. Yet, I did. I no longer view depression and anxiety with a clinician's indifferent eye, but with the sensitivity of one who knows what it feels like to be so sad it hurts or too afraid to move. The growth process during menopause was

ACHIEVING GOOD MENTAL HEALTH DURING MENOPAUSE

more painful to me than it was during my adolescence. But the message here is I survived it. And, not only did I remain sane, I became a stronger, more accepting and happier human being.

Menopause in itself was not the reason for my becoming an emotionally healthier, more relaxed person. I had to learn many coping skills to survive this period, most of which I've already shared with you. If I had to sum them up, these helping skills would fall into four major categories:

1. Nutrition, diet and vitamins
2. Exercise and other means of stress reduction
3. Hormone replacement therapy (HRT)
4. General appearance and well-being

Swede and Jaffe include diet, relaxation and exercise as part of their 7-step panic reduction program, all consistent with improved mental health during menopause. HRT and enhanced well-being are also important factors that need further discussion.

1. Nutrition. There are lots of do nots. Don't smoke, drink alcohol excessively, eat chocolate, drink caffeine. In other words, stay away from stimulants. Also try not to use products that contain aspartame that can make you nervous and depressed. Do eat a low fat diet with plenty fruits and vegetables that are loaded with natural vitamins. Soy products are great estrogen boosters if you can get past the taste. I never could. Drink water, preferably bottled. Don't hesitate to take vitamin supplements. Calcium is a must. My gynecologist recommends around 1200 mg. a day. Calcium has calming properties. A glass of milk before bedtime can do wonders in helping you get to sleep. Take vitamin E especially if you're not using estrogen and don't forget B Complex. B Complex is often recommended to reduce anxiety and stress. Talk with your doctor or pharmacist about how much E and B Complex you need. Both are good for you in general and you may be getting them in your daily multivitamin which is a must. Limit sugar and salt intake both which can stress the body. Remember to eat healthy for optimum health, both physical and emotional.

2. Exercise and other means of stress reduction. We all know that

HOW TO SURVIVE MENOPAUSE
WITHOUT GOING CRAZY

physical exercise is good for us. Exercising releases endorphins that increase our sense of well-being. Exercise also helps us feel less nervous because it reduces muscle tension. So, knowing all this, you still hate to exercise or you feel too tired to do anything physical. Remind yourself that if you force yourself to get out and take that little walk in the sunshine, you are going to be less depressed, less tense, more energetic. I mention walking because it is one of the safest, easiest forms of exercise available to us. But, the key to exercising is finding something that interests and is fun for you. Learn how to swim or try water aerobics. Take up golf or tennis. Perhaps biking appeals to you. Weight lifting is another possibility for those of us who are worried about osteoporosis. Gardening provides good exercise. A formal aerobics or dance class, even classes in square-dancing or perhaps ballroom dancing might be just what you need if you want company while you exercise. Anyway, whatever you choose, don't overdo it. If there is a physical reason for your inactivity, discuss appropriate activities with your physician. Exercise your mind to reduce stress and anxiety. There are many imaging tapes on the market to help you relax. Take deep breaths from your diaphragm several times during the day. Laughter is a great healer, so focus on watching the sitcoms on TV or checking out comedies at the video stores. A good romantic comedy always lifts my spirits. There are a couple of mental exercises I learned when dealing with panic attacks that are very helpful. One is called self-talk. It's simply telling yourself positive things about your situation when you're feeling down. For instance, when you think everyone is noticing your hot flash and you get even more anxious, you might say to yourself, "So, even if someone does see me turn red, who cares? Chances are he or she won't know what's going on. It's not a big deal. It's going to go away in a little while." Another mental exercise I found helpful was to focus on something other than that hot flash or how awful I was feeling. So, refocus. Eat something fun, talk with someone, read, count, whatever. Just refocus your attention away from the problem. Have I mentioned prayer? Whatever form prayer takes for you, indulge in it. Even if it provides little more than

ACHIEVING GOOD MENTAL HEALTH
DURING MENOPAUSE

a means to refocus, prayer helps. I have a page from a calendar in a place where I can see it everyday. I don't know who wrote it. It reads:

> "Sunlight is healing;
> fresh air is cleansing.
> When we think enough of ourselves
> to take a walk when
> we need it, even
> that small amount of self-consideration is
> healing."

3. Hormone replacement therapy (HRT). Even in the late 90's the questions about the safety of taking estrogen remain. Study after study showing the benefits and dangers of HRT have been released, each one more confusing than the other. The message is always the same. Every woman needs to decide for herself if she is a candidate for hormone replacement. Because I have a family history of heart problems, osteoporosis, and colon cancer with no history of breast cancer, the decision for me was not as difficult as it is for others. I choose to take estrogen. However, I don't want to take Provera. Provera is a progestin that is given along with estrogen to prevent a uterine lining build-up that is thought to lead to cancer. I need to take Provera since I still have a uterus. Women who have had hysterectomies don't have to worry about developing uterine cancer and can take estrogen alone or unopposed as it's called when given this way. Provera causes PMS-type symptoms for me and others who take it and also causes break-through bleeding so I'm just waiting for the day when a designer estrogen that doesn't require Provera use with it becomes available. There is talk of such a product being available in the near future. I, like most women who are perimenopausal or post-menopausal, have weighed the pros and cons of HRT. The pros far outnumber the cons. Estrogen: a. Helps memory. Prevents Alzheimers. b. Prevents heart attacks. c. May prevent colon cancer. d. Reduces hot

HOW TO SURVIVE MENOPAUSE
WITHOUT GOING CRAZY

flashes. e. Decreases blood pressure. f. Relieves other bothersome symptoms of menopause such as vaginal dryness, incontinence. I believe estrogen also does a lot of things to enhance our well-being during and after menopause that the drug companies don't lay claim to. But women taking estrogen will tell you they feel better emotionally, are less moody, sleep better, have fewer wrinkles, better sex lives. I know I could not have survived menopause without my little patch. Besides the side effects mentioned earlier, the biggest obstacle to taking HRT is the possibility that estrogen causes breast cancer. Maybe. Studies are still too inconclusive to help much in the decision of whether or not to take estrogen. If I had a family history of breast cancer I certainly would not risk taking it. Hopefully, designer estrogen is just around the corner and will be available for every woman without risk.

4. General appearance and well-being. There is nothing more vital to good mental health than feeling good about how you look. If you are a little down, get dressed, put on some make-up and you'll start to feel better. Menopause and aging, unfortunately, do coincide. I felt awful when I developed a double chin even though I was not overweight. I ordered one of these chin gym things. I still use it. I don't even know if it works. It doesn't matter. I'm doing something to enhance my looks. I'm not giving in to the so-called ravages of time. I won't age without a fight. I know several people who have already made several trips to their cosmetic surgeons before any signs of aging appears. One dealt with menopause by having boob enhancement, a face lift, vein surgery and liposuction. She absolutely refuses to "give in" to the aging process. I wish I had the guts to brave the surgeon's scalpel, but I don't. Still there are less drastic measures we can take. Find an all-day spa and indulge in a new hairstyle or color, a manicure or pedicure. Let someone treat you to a therapeutic massage. Go shopping for a whole new wardrobe to fit the trimmer, firmer you after all that exercise. Get dressed up and go out with someone you really like or who's fun to be with. I found associating with other menopausal women really helped. Especially close friends and family. If

ACHIEVING GOOD MENTAL HEALTH DURING MENOPAUSE

I was having dinner with such a person and had a hot-flash with a resulting panic attack as the adrenalin surged through my body, I could just say so and I knew that my companion would understand. Sometimes my friends and I shared our hot flashes and we could actually laugh about what was happening to us. I didn't need a formal support group because my sisters and several friends experienced perimenopause at the same time I did. Don't go through menopause alone. Your husband and children will try to help, but they don't really understand what it's like to go through these often traumatic changes. Find a group of women who are currently experiencing menopause to help you get through it. I learned so much from my own little circle of menopausal friends and family about what to expect and what worked and what didn't to relieve symptoms of menopause and make me look and feel better.

In a recent article in *Prevention* magazine, Dr. Brian Walsh, M.D. informed readers that "80% of women report some kind of disturbance of mood or thinking." It is so gratifying to have that fact acknowledged. I think we'd all like to believe that most women breeze through menopause without any emotional problems, but we are doing a disservice to all women if we don't prepare them for the reality of the situation. We can do this without frightening them. It's scary enough when young women see their mothers go through some of these emotional changes and not know what's happening. Courage is found in knowledge. When a mother who has just delivered a baby knows she can expect to feel a little blue for a few days, she will not be frightened by what is happening to her. The same goes for women about to enter perimenopause.

We have talked about a lot of symptoms that make up the emotional component of menopause. Luckily, most women will experience only one or two of them. Some will be nervous and tense. Others may feel a little blue and suffer from mood swings. Still others may have insomnia and be irritable and impatient the following day. Some may feel fatigued and have trouble concentrating. A few will have that creepy-crawly feeling that I found so weird. But, most all of us will be afraid sometime during this

HOW TO SURVIVE MENOPAUSE
WITHOUT GOING CRAZY

perimenopause phase of the change. Hopefully, not one woman who is prepared for what happens during a hot flash will develop extreme anxiety and panic attacks as I did. You know one of the things that can happen during a panic attack is the feeling that you're losing your mind. It was the scariest thing about having one as far as I am concerned.

Not only do we hope to emerge from menopause sane or emotionally intact, we need to try to achieve good mental health during this difficult period of out lives. The challenges after menopause are plentiful and we need to be equipped for further growth. When we retire from our jobs and go back to college or seek out other intellectual or professional pursuits. And especially, for those wonderful years when we begin to welcome a new generation into our hearts and lives. When our children's children arrive just in time to teach us how to be young again.

BIBLIOGRAPHY

Burnett, Raymond G., M.D. Menopause: All Your Questions Answered. Chicago: Contemporary Books, Inc., 1987.

Cutler, Winnifred B., Ph.D. and Ramon Garcia Celso, M.D. Menopause: A Guide For Women and the Men Who Love Them. New York: W.W. Norton and Co., 1983, Revised, 1992.

Dranov, Paula. Estrogen: Is It Right for You? New York: Simon and Schuster, 1993.

English, O. Spurgeon, M.D. and Gerald H.J. Pearson, M.D. Emotional Problems of Living: Avoiding the Neurotic Pattern. New York: W.W. Norton and Co., 1945, Revised 1963.

Fergerson, Tom, M.D. The No-Nag No-Guilt Do-It-Your-Own-Way Guide to Quitting Smoking. New York: Ballantine Books, 1987.

Gitlin, M.J. and R.O. Pasnau. "Psychiatric Syndromes Linked to Reproductive Function in Women: A Review of Current Knowledge." American Journal of Psychiatry. 146:11, 1989.

Greenwood, Sadja, M.D. Menopause Naturally: Preparing for the Second Half of Life. San Francisco: Volvano Press, 1984.

Greer, Germaine. The Change: Women, Aging and the Menopause. New York: Alfred A. Knoph, 1992.

Henkel, Gretchen. Making the Estrogen Decision. Los Angeles: Lowell House, 1992.

Higbee, Kenneth L., Ph.D. Your Memory: How It Works and How to Improve It. New York: Paragon House, 1993.

HOW TO SURVIVE MENOPAUSE
WITHOUT GOING CRAZY

Nachttigal, Lila, M.D. and John Rahner Heilman. Estrogen: The Facts Can Change Your Life. New York: Harper and Row, 1986.

National Institution Aging. The Menopause Time of Life. NHI Publication 86-2461, July, 1986.

Sheehy, Gail. The Silent Passage: Menopause. New York: Random House, 1992.

Swede, Shirley and Seymour Sheppard Jaffe, M.D. The Panic Attack Recovery Book. New York: Signet, 1989.

U.S. Congress, Office of Technology Assessment. The Menopause Hormone Therapy and Women's Health. OTA-BP-BA-88. Washington, DC: U.S. Government Printing Office, May, 1992.

Utian, Wulf H., M.D., Ph.D. and Ruth S. Jacobowitz. Managing Your Menopause. New York: Prentice Hall Press, 1990.

Vliet, Elizabeth Lee, M.D. and Virginia Lee Hutcheson Davis, M.S. "New Perspectives on the Relationship of Hormone Changes to Affective Disorders in the Perimenopause." NAACOG'S Clinical Issues Vol 2 No 4, 1991.

Author's Note

The controversy regarding hormone replacement therapy (HRT) remains the same since this book was first published in the late 1990's. Recent studies still show a slight increase in the occurrence of breast cancer for those of us using HRT, but there are several new alternatives to HRT available for the treatment of osteoporosis, etc.

If I were to rename this book, I'd call it, How To Survive Perimenopause Without Going Crazy, since it is during these five to ten years before menopause that hormones fluctuate and emotions rage. One thing remains certain, we can survive menopause without going crazy.

From the other side of menopause,

Leona Lipari Lee

Fall, 2001

e-mail me at mvllll@swbell.net

Printed in the United States
23368LVS00006B/1